Yoga and Pilates for your Mind, Body and Baby

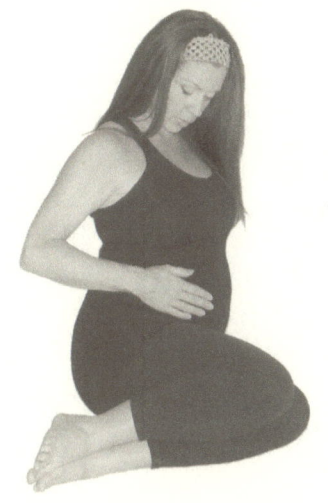

Lisa T. Daniel

AuthorHouse™
1663 Liberty Drive
Bloomington, IN 47403
www.authorhouse.com
Phone: 1-800-839-8640

First published by AuthorHouse 8/11/2010

ISBN: 978-1-4490-8074-7 (sc)
ISBN: 978-1-4490-8075-4 (e)

Library of Congress Control Number: 2010923965
Printed in the United States of America
Bloomington, Indiana

This book is printed on acid-free paper.

Edited by: Vance Ledford

Before practicing "Yoga and Pilates for your Mind, Body and Baby", it is recommended that you first check with your doctor or health care provider. Although this material has been prepared with care, the Publisher does not accept responsibility for injury to any person as a result of participation in this program.

DEDICATION

I dedicate this book to my baby girl Nina. Her presence in my life has made me realize how precious life really is. Everyday has taken on new meaning and purpose, and it is she who has been my inspiration.

Nina has created within me a need to share my knowledge and expertise with all the future mothers out there, and I feel her coming into my life has been a blessing, not only to me, but to all the women out there who are also inspired by my teachings.

ACKNOWLEDGMENT

There are many people out there who have helped to make this book possible. First I'd like to thank my baby girl Nina. Her arrival into my life has been my true inspiration.

I would also like to thank my mother Agnes whose unconditional love throughout my entire life has helped make all this possible. My father, Normand, also deserves many thanks for all of his positive words of encouragement and for his strength and discipline which he so strongly instilled within me. My two wonderful sisters Diana and Linda I must thank for always being there and inspiring me to do and be my best.

I would like to thank Vance Ledford for being my friend and business confidant. His expertise was crucial in bringing this book and its companion DVD to reality. Also, I would like to thank Karla Bradis for her help, and for introducing me to Vance.

Lastly, I thank all of my close friends who have been positive influences and who helped to make this happen by being such supportive and loving friends.

CONTENTS

Mountain Pose, Chest Expansion, Side Bend Stretch,
Squats & Plie Squats, Yoga Mudra, Arm Circles, Genie
Arm Twists, Pilates One Foot Balance, Tree Pose,
Straddle Splits, Squat and Rise Pose

Cat/Cow Pose, Spinal Balancing with Leg Lifts, Pelvic
Circles, Child's Pose, Lunge, Striking Cobra Pose,
Downward Facing Dog Pose, Plank Pose

CONTENTS (cont.)

INTRODUCTION

Yoga & Pilates for your Mind Body and Baby has been created to help you get the most out of your pregnancy by providing you with the safest forms of exercise. These poses and exercises will allow the best physical and emotional environment for both you and your baby. You will learn Yoga and Pilates as well as breathing techniques and their benefits in detail. All of these techniques are meant to be performed slowly and gently. They are all safe and effective for all levels of pregnancy unless otherwise noted. Your strength, balance and flexibility will be enhanced while the stress and aches and pains of pregnancy may be eliminated. These gentle movements will also provide you with increased stamina which will prepare you for labor and childbirth and beyond.

You will find that the same principals that are applied to Yoga and Pilates will also apply here, however the poses and exercises have been modified to accommodate you and your ever-changing body. There will be many physical as well as emotional changes and challenges throughout your pregnancy. Some of these changes may seem overwhelming at times, resulting in a lack of confidence or control.

Yoga and Pilates for your Mind Body and Baby will give you the tools to help you manage your mind and body during this great time of change. These movements will allow you to feel peaceful and calm within as they bring more balance back into your life physically as well as emotionally. These movements will bring stress relief as they allow your hormone levels to shift and rebalance themselves. Deep breathing, which is encouraged throughout, allows more oxygen to all of the muscles in your body, thereby promoting more relaxation as well as creating more room for your baby in your belly.

When practiced regularly, you will feel the mental and physical benefits of this routine. You will approach each day feeling a little better and more positive about yourself! You will become more in tune with your body and with the wonderful miracle of your baby growing within your belly. This is the perfect way to honor and nurture yourself... your mind, your body and your baby!

PRECAUTIONS

Prior to beginning Yoga and Pilates during your pregnancy, you should consult your doctor or health care professional to be sure that you don't have any conditions that could prevent you from participating. If your doctor has given you the go ahead then enjoy this book and my DVD as well.

Allow modifications to your movements as your body changes, giving you more flexibility to continue with the program. It is important to know the limitations of your body at all times and to honor them. Do not push yourself to a place that does not feel comfortable for you. Take your time and have an awareness of your breathing throughout. The breath will help you to relax more fully into your movements.

Avoid all movements where your head is below your heart if you are experiencing high or low blood pressure. Also, if Yoga and Pilates are new for you, then it is not recommended that you do forward bends or inverted poses during your Third Trimester. If you feel any discomfort or strain in the abdomen at any time then discontinue the movement. Remember, these movements are meant to be gentle on your body.

Lying on your back for an extended period of time can feel uncomfortable for some women due to the weight and pressure of your abdomen on the vena cava. The vena cava is a major artery on the right side of your body. Listen to your body and discontinue that particular movement if needed.

If at any time you feel tired, are struggling or have shortness of breath, then please back out of the movement and return to breathing deeply and slowly. This will help restore your energy levels and bring a sense of calm back into your body.

Lastly, be sure to always listen closely to your body. Have awareness at every moment of your breath, your emotions and all physical sensations. These movements are meant to be gentle without any strain or discomfort to you. They are meant to be experienced with joy and oneness as you meld together that miraculous connection of your mind, your body and your baby!

HEALTHY EATING

Good nutrition is very important during pregnancy.
You want to eat smart and make healthy choices. You
really only need an extra 300 calories a day to support
your baby's growth and development. You want to choose
foods from each of the five food groups as they will
provide you with the essential nutrients that both you and
your baby will need.

Grains, Fruits, Vegetables, Dairy and Proteins are
your five food groups to choose from. Six to ten servings
of grains and breads per day, four or more servings of
veggies per day, two to four servings of fruits per day,
four or more servings of dairy products per day and three
servings of proteins a day is recommended during your
pregnancy. Be careful with the sweets and the fats. Use
them sparingly.

Choose foods that are high in fiber such as whole-
grain breads, cereals, wheat pasta, brown rice, fruits and
vegetables.

Eat and drink at least four servings of dairy products
and calcium-rich foods a day to help you get enough
calcium. Such sources are milk, yogurt, natural cheese
such as cheddar or processed cheese such as American.

Eat at least three servings of iron-rich foods per day
to ensure you are getting 27 mg of iron daily. Lean meats,
poultry, fish and nuts are healthy choices.

Choose a good source of Vitamin C every day such as
oranges, cantaloupe, papaya, strawberries, honeydew,
kiwifruit, broccoli, brussel sprouts, peppers and tomatoes.

Good sources of Vitamin A every day include carrots,
pumpkins, sweet potatoes, spinach, water squash, turnip
greens, beet greens, apricots, cantaloupe, peaches,
papayas and mangos.

Folic Acid is very important during your pregnancy.
Folic acid is a form of the B vitamin that aids in the
regular cellular development and regeneration of your
baby. Good sources include dark green leafy vegetables,
beans, lentils, chickpeas, chicken or beef liver and

breakfast cereals. Other sources include oatmeal, aspara-
gus, spinach and romaine lettuce.

Be sure to get a good prenatal vitamin from your
doctor or ask what over the counter prenatal supplements
he or she recommends for you.

FOODS TO AVOID

While dieting is definitely not recommended during
pregnancy, a healthy balanced diet is essential. Both you
and your baby need the proper nutrients in order to be
healthy. Obviously some of the foods that you will crave
during your pregnancy may not be all that good for you.
Making healthy choices over unhealthy ones is the best
you can do for yourself and your baby. The more knowledge you have, the more equipped you will be to make
the best possible choices.

High Fat foods- Good fat is especially vital to your
baby, particularly when it comes to Omega-3 fatty acids,
which fuel proper brain growth and eye development.
Unnecessary fats such as sugary and salty junk food
contain empty, unhealthy calories with no nutritional
value. Unnecessary fats can also increase your child's risk
of obesity, overeating, diabetes and heart disease in the
future. Eating junk food can actually cause your baby to
develop a taste for junk food, making it more difficult for
them to make healthy eating choices in the future.

Raw Meats, Eggs and Seafood including Sushi - All
uncooked and rare meats, eggs and seafood run a high
risk of listeria and/or salmonella poisoning and must be
avoided. Avoid foods made with raw or partially cooked
eggs. Such things may be eggnog, Caesar salad dressing
and hollandaise sauce.

Deli meats including hot dogs - Deli meats might be
contaminated with listeria bacteria. It's safe to eat deli
meats if you reheat them until steaming hot.

Refrigerated smoked seafood, refrigerated pâté or meat spreads – Avoid these for the same reason of listeria contamination. It is safe if they are contained in cooked dishes. Canned and shelf-stable versions are safe to eat.

Fish high in mercury - Avoid high-mercury fish such as Shark, Swordfish, King Mackerel and Tilefish. Shellfish, such as oysters and clams can be high in bacteria. Also tropical fish, such as Mahi - Mahi and Grouper may also have some toxins that are not safe.

Soft cheese - Avoid the following soft cheeses: Feta, Brie and Camembert cheeses, blue-veined cheeses, queso blanco, queso fresco and Panela. They are safe to eat if they are labeled pasteurized.

Liver -Liver is a rich source of iron. However it contains a high level of Vitamin A. Large amounts of Vitamin A can be harmful to the baby.

Unpasteurized milk, smoothies, yogurts and juices- Be sure to check the labels to see if they are pasteurized.

Alcohol and Caffeine - Caffeine and alcohol can prevent absorption of folic acid and iron. These nutrients are essential during pregnancy. They also directly affect the fetus and can have long-term developmental effects. A healthy limit of caffeine would be no more than 300 mg per day. An 8-ounce cup of coffee has about 150 mg of caffeine. Sodas, teas and chocolate contain caffeine as well, so watch these closely.

Sprouts- Avoid alfalfa and wheat sprouts as they may be contaminated with bacteria like E. coli.

Unwashed Fruits and Vegetables- Make sure all vegetables are washed to avoid potential exposure to toxoplasmosis. Toxoplasmosis is a parasitic disease caused by a parasite that may be present in the soil where the fruits and vegetables are grown.

WHAT YOU WILL NEED

Everything that you will need you will more than likely already have at home.

For starters, find a **comfortable temperature** you can work within. A warm environment can assist a gentle workout, but it is important that the body not be made to hot or too cold. Extremes in temperature, especially heat, can have negative affects on the body.

Water is a very important part of your pregnancy and acts as the body's transportation system, carrying nutrients through your blood to your baby. Also, flushing out your system and diluting your urine with water helps to prevent urinary tract infections, which are common during pregnancy. Perhaps the most important reason to drink water however is to keep your body hydrated. Dehydration can be a serious thing. Hormones will change the way you store water during your pregnancy resulting more often than not in the retention of water. Drinking plenty of water helps to combat that. It is also highly recommended that you drink water regularly to prevent your body from over-heating. Drink 8 ounces of water 20-30 minutes prior to exercise and 8 ounces every 20 minutes during exercise.

Always wear **loose clothes** to prevent discomfort and overheating. The more comfortable you feel the more likely you will enjoy the routine and stick with it.

A **yoga mat** will be most beneficial to do your movements on. You may also want a few pillows to provide you with extra support as well as a small and/or large rolled up towel. A block is optional but may be helpful in forward movements to reach the ground better. A strap or belt of some kind that is comfortable to hold is also recommended.

Lastly, I would recommend **a chair** if you are practicing these movements during your Third Trimester and feel that your balance may be compromised. A chair can help you to maintain some of the standing postures more effectively.

BREATHING

The greatest tool to help you find peace and relaxation will come through your breath. When you become in tune with the natural rhythms of your breath you become aware, deeply aware, of a connectedness and oneness with your mind and your body.

Deep breathing during pregnancy is a must. It can help in elimination of stress and anxiety. In addition, abdominal breathing can help you deal with the physical discomforts of pregnancy, such as labor and delivery.

Deep breathing exercises help in passing more oxygen to the blood, to the brain, and to all of the muscles in your body being utilized throughout these movements.

It is very useful to control stress and irritation, and it helps brings back focus and concentration into your life. More importantly, the breath prepares you for birth!!

Deep breathing isn't something we are accustomed to doing. It takes regular practice. When you breathe deeply it is coming from the abdomen and diaphragm.

HOW TO PRACTICE DEEP BREATHING

To practice deep breathing, lie on your mat with your knees bent, your feet hip distance width apart and your arms relaxed by your sides. If in this position you feel any neck strain then place a small towel or pillow beneath your neck for support. Begin to notice your breathing... your natural flow of breath. Take notice whether your chest is rising and falling or your belly... or maybe it is both. Notice if there is tension in these areas and relax them. Try now to breathe in through your rib cage.

To breathe more effectively the aim is to send the breath into the back of the rib cage which expands the rib cage outwardly or laterally on each inhalation.

Begin by bringing your hands to the base of your rib cage placing your fingers on the front of your lower ribs and your thumbs on the back of your rib cage. Breathe in through your nose as you guide your breath down toward the bottom and back of your rib cage expanding it wide from side to side... almost like an accordion. Your abdomen should move outward as you inhale. If only your chest is moving, then you aren't inhaling deeply enough. Then exhale through your mouth and actively pull your rib bones inward and close together. Practice this a few moments. Repeat several times, working up to about 10 breaths to be sure you fully feel this movement.

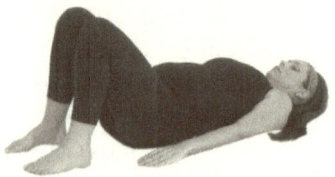

Your exhalation is also very important, just as important as your inhalation. The exhalation allows for a deepening of the lower abdominal musculature. Inhale into the sides and back of your rib cage and then as you exhale flatten your abdomen by imagining you are drawing your navel to your spine. Inhale again to expand the rib cage and exhale through the mouth while drawing your navel deeper and deeper in towards your spine and then relax. Now place your fingertips gently on your navel centre. Continue to breathe in as you expand your ribs laterally and now as you exhale and draw your navel toward your spine try to actually draw your navel away from your fingertips creating space between the two. Try this for a few breaths as well.

As your belly grows you may find abdominal breathing becomes more difficult for you as your growing uterus presses upward against your ribs and diaphragm. Do your best to breathe as deeply as you can. This can only help both you and your baby benefit from the additional oxygen and the relaxation it brings. It is common to feel dizzy or faint when beginning to breathe in this manner. If you are feeling these symptoms then try to slow down your breathing, or rest for a moment or two before beginning again.

NEUTRAL PELVIS

You will find that it will be beneficial to you to understand a neutral pelvis to get the most out of this routine. Neutral pelvis is the positioning of your pelvis that is most natural and normal for proper body mechanics to take place. This position preserves the slight, natural curves of the spine, especially the low back, and allows your abdominals to engage more effectively.

HOW TO PRACTICE NEUTRAL PELVIS

To practice Neutral Pelvis in the lying down position, lie on your back with knees bent, feet flat and about hip width apart. Place your hands on your lower abdominals. Inhale, then exhale and draw your belly button into your low back, so much that you gently press your low back down into the mat, rocking your hips towards your face. Your buttocks will not actually leave the floor, but you will feel your low back press into the floor. You are essentially taking the curve out of the low back.

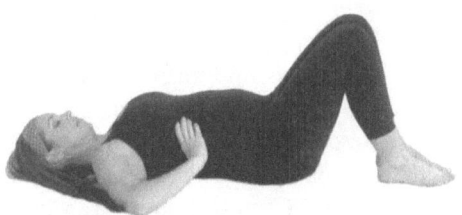

Inhale and release your belly button so you lower back lifts out of the floor and slightly arches off the mat and then exhale again as you flatten out your back. Go back and forth between these two positions so you can get a feel for them. It may feel as if you are rocking like a seesaw back and forth. Know that neither of these two extremes is considered a neutral pelvis. Stop the movement now and settle at a place between these two extremes. Find a comfortable position that feels centered and feels natural to you.

You should still have a small natural arch in your back but not quite enough to get your fingers under. Relax, and get the feel of neutral pelvis into your mind.

To practice Neutral Pelvis in a seated position, sit on a block or a stool so you can feel your sits bones. These are the bones that you feel beneath you when you sit up straight. Feel the length from your sits bones through the top of your head.

Take a deep breath and close your eyes to bring more awareness to what you are feeling. Feel the length from your sits bones through the top of your head. Notice the length of your spine all the way up. Begin by slowly tipping your pelvis forward. Stop when you begin to feel the lower back harden, which will be a natural result of the back muscles shortening and tightening.

Bring the pelvis back upright and slowly tip the pelvis back in the opposite direction until you feel the abdominals harden. The movement, as you will see, will not be a large one in either direction.

Your neutral position once again is somewhere between these two places where both the abdominals and the back are soft and not gripping or feeling tight or constricted in any way at all.

Practice this a few times and notice that when you are in a neutral position you can feel your sits bones grounded firmly and your torso in perfect alignment without any stress on your body or muscles at all.

You should still have a small natural arch in your back but not quite enough to get your fingers under. Relax, and get the feel of neutral pelvis into your mind.

PELVIC FLOOR EXERCISES

Pelvic floor exercises can help strengthen your pelvic floor muscles which support the uterus, bladder and bowel. The more you use them the stronger they will be. The pelvic floor is the muscle group that controls the flow of urine and the contraction of the vagina and the anal sphincter. These muscles play a very important role in maintaining general health throughout your life and proper functioning of the entire pelvic region.

When your pelvic floor muscles weaken, your pelvic organs drop downward and bulge into your vagina. This is known as pelvic organ prolapse. This can result in uncomfortable pelvic pressure as well as leakage of urine or feces. Fortunately, pelvic floor exercises can strengthen pelvic muscles and delay or even prevent pelvic organ prolapse. It is therefore essential to exercise these muscles regularly and keep them as firm as possible.

Having a toned pelvic floor will help your body deal with supporting the weight of your growing baby as well as enable your pelvic floor muscle to recover more quickly after the birth of your baby. The wonderful thing about doing these exercises is that they can be done virtually anywhere.

To know where they are first of all, try to stop the flow of urine while you're going to the bathroom. If you succeed, you've got the basic feeling. Don't make a habit of starting and stopping your urine stream as this can actually weaken the muscles. It can also lead to incomplete emptying of the bladder, which increases your risk of urinary tract infections.

Once you've identified your pelvic floor muscles, empty your bladder and lie down.

HOW TO PRACTICE PELVIC FLOOR EXERCISES

Take a deep breath. As you exhale, contract your pelvic floor by drawing your tailbone toward your pubic bone. Do this without moving your pelvis.

Think about trying to keep from passing gas. Hold the

contraction for at least three seconds and up to ten seconds while you are exhaling. Relax for the same amount of time and repeat the process.

Be careful not to flex or move the muscles in your pelvic area. Also, try not to hold your breath. Just relax, breathe freely and focus on tightening the muscles between your tailbone toward your pubic bone. Do not strain down but instead draw the muscles up and inward.

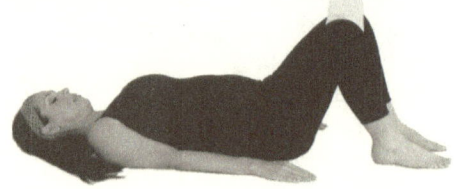

If you cannot feel the contraction, bring your knees up and try squeezing a pillow between your knees while exhaling and contracting the pelvic floor. Remember, the contraction does not require a lot of force - just enough to turn the muscles on and keep them on for up to ten seconds and release. Inhale to prepare. Then exhale and squeeze the pillow without movement in your pelvis. Imagine you are holding the flow of urine. Try to contract only the pelvic muscles. (If you feel your abdomen, thighs or buttocks tightening then relax, remove the pillow and aim just for the pelvic muscles by using a less intense muscle contraction.)

Perform a set of ten, three times a day. The more you practice the easier this will become. Try contracting the muscles in many different positions such as standing upright, lying, sitting, on hands and knees, feet together and feet apart. See which way feels most effective to you.

SPINAL ALIGNMENT

During pregnancy, our spinal alignment or posture can become challenged. Specific muscles can become too tight and others overstretched, causing stress to our physical bodies and our overall well-being. Being aware of this, and through practice, we can help to maintain more balance in our bodies.

Due to the weight of our belly, there can often be a tilt in the pelvis resulting in a tightening of the hips as well as an overstretching and weakening of the hamstrings or back of the thighs. Because of the belly size your abdominal muscles are overstretched and weakened. Your weight, as a result, tends to shift towards the balls of your feet, which in turn tightens the calve muscles. The lower back muscles are normally affected as well and the lower back muscle will shorten, tighten and may cause pain.

The increased size of the breasts tends to pull the shoulders forward, which shortens and tightens your chest muscles. When the shoulders round and the chest tightens, normally there will be a forward shifting of the head which tightens the neck muscles. By stretching the muscles that have become tight and by strengthening the muscles which have become weak, you will achieve improved balance, coordination, and posture during all nine months of your pregnancy and after.

HOW TO PRACTICE SPINAL ALIGNMENT

Begin by bringing your pelvis back into a neutral position. This will open the hips and allow the hamstrings to shift back to normal length. Your back muscles will also lengthen and relax. Shift your weight back into your heels releasing your overstretched calves. Open the chest and roll your shoulders back and down which lengthens your chest muscle and strengthens your upper back. As a result your head will shift back over your shoulders in a neutral position, releasing and relaxing your neck muscles.

Stretching in this way as well as strengthening will improve your physical well being as well as your emotional health. The stretching will help to align and center your spine at the same time allowing you to feel more mentally centered and calm.

FIRST & SECOND TRIMESTER EXERCISES/POSES

STANDING POSES

MOUNTAIN POSE

Benefits: This pose helps to align the spine, improve the posture and develop physical and mental balance. The muscles of the feet and legs will strengthen as a result of balancing on the toes. The abdominal muscles will also feel strengthened as well as lengthened. This posture also helps with developing more focus and concentration, thereby relieving anxiety.

1. Stand with the feet hip width apart and hold a strap loosely in your hands (fig.1). Focus straight ahead at eye level.

2. Inhale to raise the arms overhead as you lift up onto the toes. Draw the shoulder blades down and away from the ears as you reach upward toward the ceiling. Balance for few moments (fig. 2).

3. Exhale and slowly begin to lower the arms while lowering the heels to the ground (fig.3). Repeat 5 times.

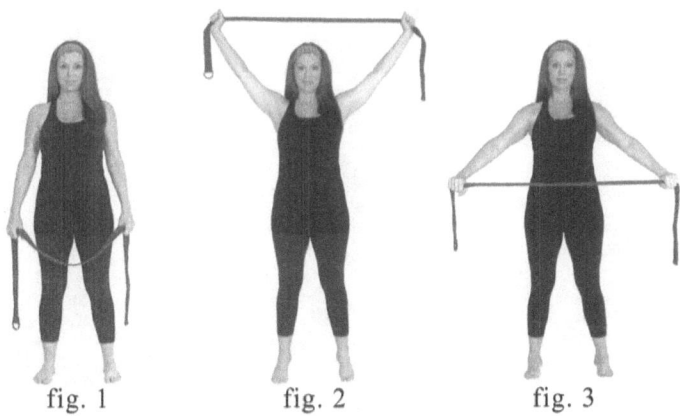

fig. 1   fig. 2   fig. 3

CHEST EXPANSION

Benefits: This pose helps to open and expand the chest area. This pose will also release tension and tightness in the upper back, shoulders and chest and will allow for better posture and breathing.

1. Stand with the feet hip width apart and hold a strap loosely in your hands (fig. 1). Focus straight ahead at eye level.

2. Inhale to raise the arms overhead and exhale to draw the shoulder blades down and away from the ears (fig.2). Inhale to extend the arms back as you stretch and open the chest area (fig. 3). Exhale to return the arms back overhead. Repeat up to 5 times.

3. Slowly lower the arms back down in front of the body.

*HINT
Be mindful of your posture and avoid arching the back as this can cause discomfort.

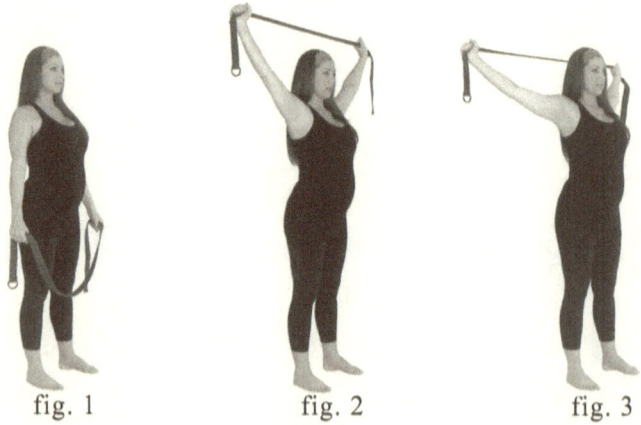

fig. 1   fig. 2   fig. 3

SIDE BEND STRETCH

Benefits: This posture helps tone the abdominal obliques and side flexors, stretches the lower back, and helps to keep the spine flexible.

1. Stand with the feet hip width apart and hold a strap loosely in your hands (fig. 1). Focus straight ahead at eye level.

2. Inhale to raise the arms overhead and exhale to draw the shoulder blades down and away from the ears (fig. 2). Exhale to extend the body over to the right (fig. 3). Inhale to return to the center (fig. 4) and exhale the body over to the left (fig. 5). Repeat up to 5 times going further into the stretch each time.

3. Return the arms to the center position and then slowly lower the arms back down in front of the body.

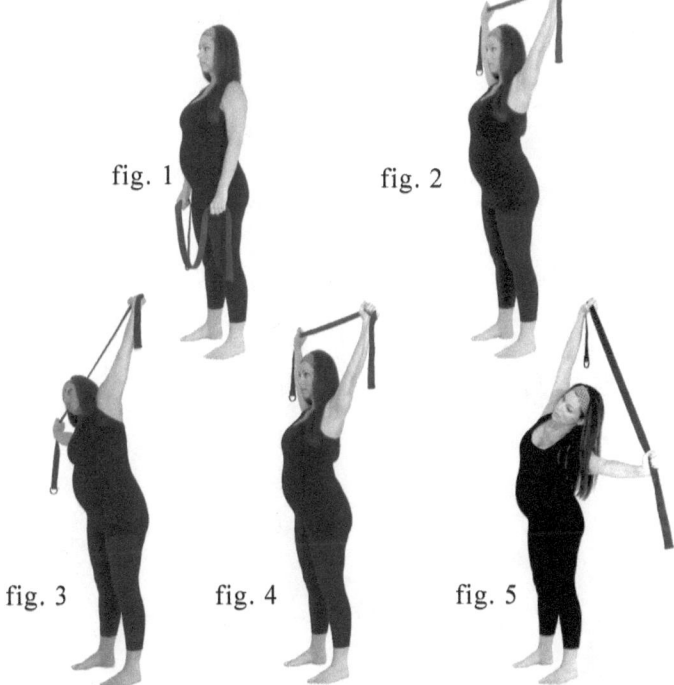

fig. 1   fig. 2

fig. 3   fig. 4   fig. 5

SQUATS & PLIE SQUATS

Benefits: This exercise helps to strengthen the pelvic floor muscles and the uterus. Squats also help encourage flexibility in the hip and the knees as well as relieve lower back discomfort and pain. Plie Squats assist in strengthening the core, the thighs and opening of the pelvis.

1. Stand with the feet hip width apart or wider and hold onto a strap loosely in the hands (fig. 1). Inhale to lift the arms to shoulder level while bending the knees and lowering the body into a squat position (fig. 2). Exhale to return to a standing posture. Repeat up to 5 times.

2. Lift up unto the toes and repeat the same movement (figs. 3 & 4). Focus on your balance as you look straight ahead at a focal point in front of you. Repeat up to 5 times.

3. Repeat steps 1 and 2 with the arms overhead (figs. 5 & 6)

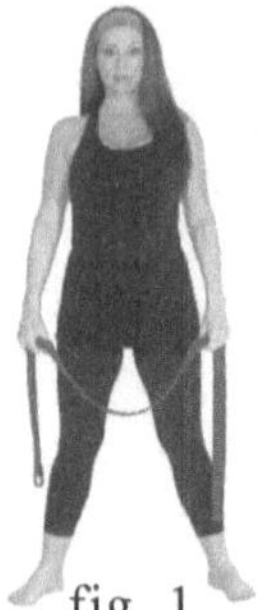

fig. 1

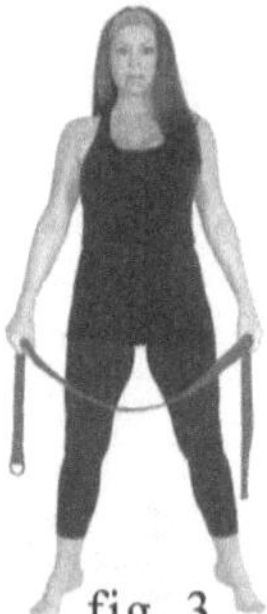

fig. 3

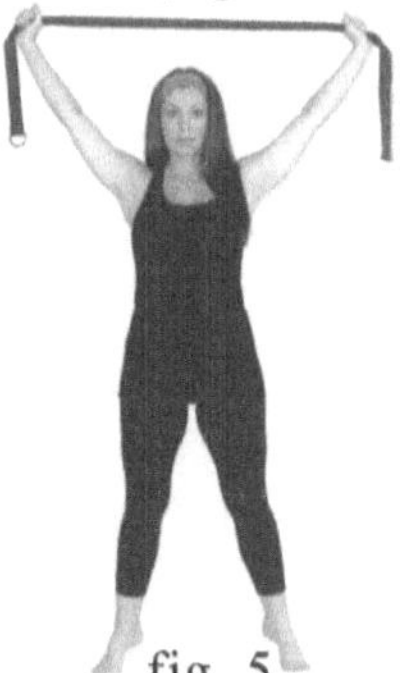

fig. 5

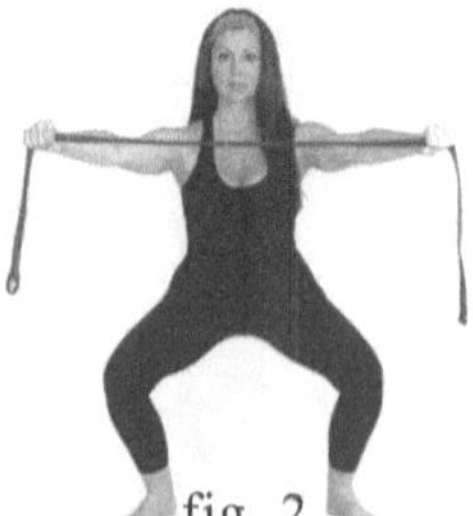

fig. 2

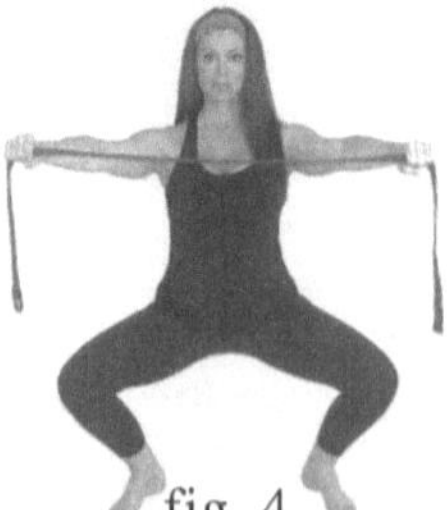

fig. 4

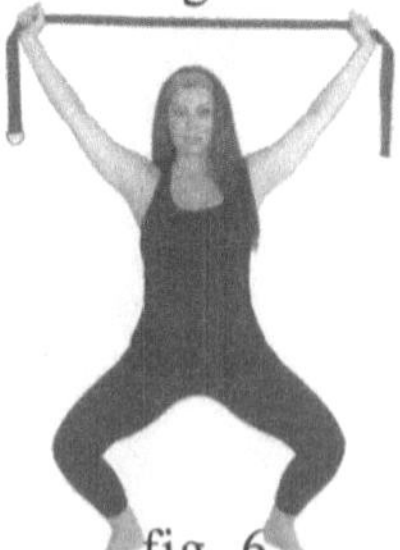

fig. 6

YOGA MUDRA

Benefits: This pose helps to strengthen the shoulder and chest muscles as well as increase their flexibility. It is a forward bend; the hamstrings will stretch as well. Yoga Mudra Pose inverts the body which greatly benefits the circulatory and immune system. Yoga Mudra also deeply calms the nervous system and the emotions.

1. Stand with the feet hip width apart. Tuck the tailbone down while engaging the core. Relax the arms straight down by your sides with the palms facing backward while holding onto a strap (fig. 1).

2. Inhale and raise the arms away from the sacrum (fig. 2) and exhale to hinge forward from the hips (fig. 3).

3. To come out of the pose, inhale again and then exhale to slowly come back to a standing position and return the arms by your sides (fig. 1). Repeat 3 to 5 times.

*HINT
Keep the knees slightly bent throughout. If you have blood pressure issues, keep the head above the heart.

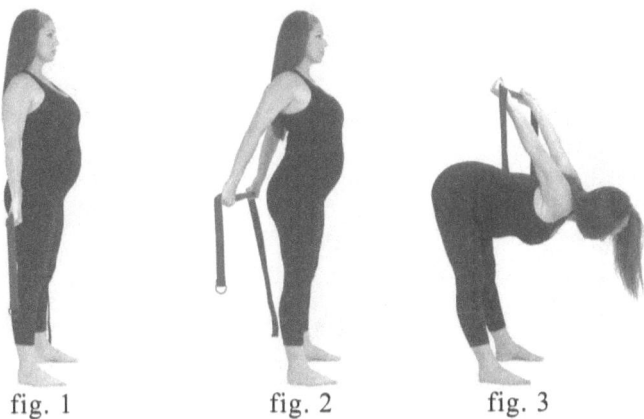

fig. 1   fig. 2   fig. 3

ARM CIRCLES

Benefits: This exercise encourages deep breathing. It improves flexibility of the shoulders and spine and provides a wonderful stretch to the sides of the body. It is also very peaceful and relaxing to the body.

1. Stand with the feet hip width apart and the palms together in front of the heart center in prayer position (fig. 1). Tuck the tailbone slightly downward while engaging the core.

2. Inhale to raise the arms overhead and stretch toward the ceiling with the fingertips allowing for a nice stretch through the sides of the body (fig. 2). Look upward and go into a very slight back-bend.

3. Exhale to reach the arms wide to the side of the room while lowering them slowly (fig. 3).

4 Return the hands to the heart center and repeat 3 to 5 times.

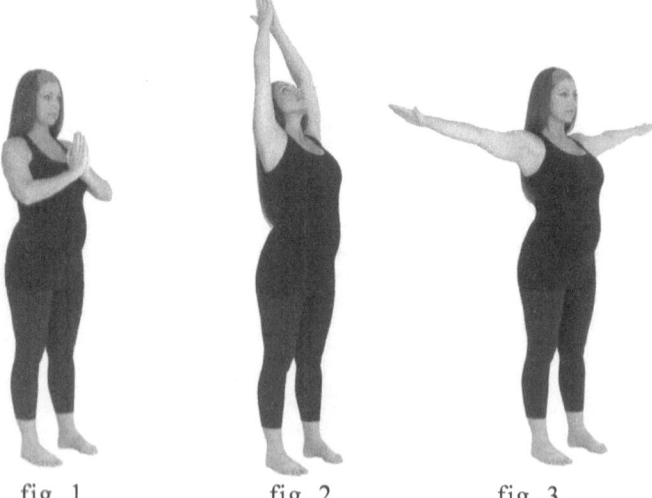

fig. 1   fig. 2   fig. 3

GENIE ARM TWIST

Benefits: This exercise stretches the muscles of the arm as well as the upper back. It also helps to release tension in the shoulders.

1. Stand with the feet hip width apart. Reach the arms out to the sides of the body (fig. 1).

2. Rotate one arm forward as the other arm rotates back (fig 2). Reach long through the fingertips and press downward with the shoulder blades.

3. Repeat in the opposite direction (fig.3) and repeat 3 to 5 times.

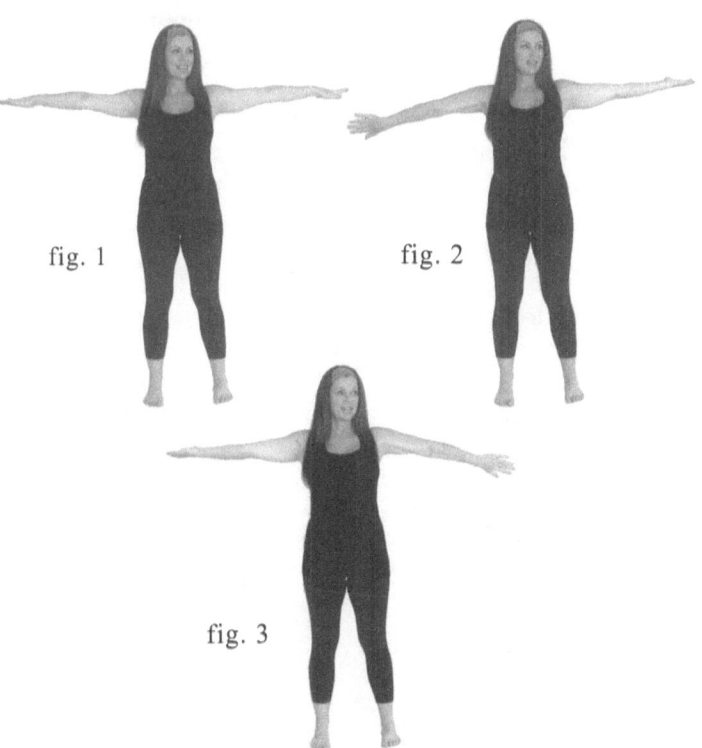

fig. 1   fig. 2

fig. 3

PILATES ONE FOOT BALANCE

Benefits: This exercise strengthens the hip, knee and ankle stabilizers as well as the thighs and buttocks. It also improves balance, focus and concentration. Pilates One Foot Balancing strengthens the core and calms and centers the mind.

1. Stand with the feet hip width apart (fig. 1). Draw the tailbone slightly downward and engage the core. Begin by shifting all of the weight to the right foot. Feel all four corners of the right foot pressing into the ground. Lift the knee cap upward toward the hip by engaging the right thigh muscle. Feel a strong line of energy from the heel up to your hip.

2. Raise both arms out to the side of the body in alignment with the shoulders with the palms pressing downward (fig. 2). Inhale the left leg up bringing the knee in alignment with the hip (fig. 3). Inhale to lower the leg touching the big toe to the ground and exhale as you engage in the pelvic floor to lift the leg back up. Repeat 5 times.

3. Extend the leg straight and then inhale to lower the straight leg toward the ground and exhale to lift the leg (fig. 4). Repeat 5 times. Switch legs.

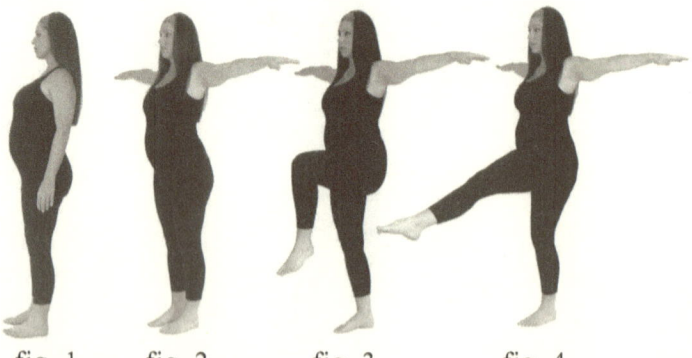

fig. 1   fig. 2   fig. 3   fig. 4

TREE POSE

Benefits: This pose helps to lengthen and strengthen the spine, improves posture, and improves physical and mental balance, focus and concentration. Tree Pose strengthens the core, legs and promotes circulation which may reduce leg cramps.

1. Stand with the feet hip width apart, tailbone aiming downward and relax the arms by your sides (fig. 1). Press evenly through the feet engaging the thigh muscles. Lift the pelvic floor muscles and engage the core. Focus at a point about 45 degrees below eye level in front of you. Shift all of the weight to the right foot and feel a strong line of energy from the heel up to your hip. Do not lock the knee.

2. Inhale and place the sole of the left foot either over the opposite ankle, higher up the leg pressing into the calf or against the inner thigh of the right leg. Exhale to relax. Bring the palms together in front of the heart in prayer position (fig. 2, next page). Press down through the right foot and reach the crown of the head up toward the ceiling.

3. Inhale the arms overhead and reach the fingertips toward the ceiling (fig. 3). Lift out of the waist feeling this wonderful stretch in your abdomen. Open your arms in a wide V for more balance (fig. 4). Hold for a few breaths. Focus on keeping the hips square and maintaining a neutral spinal alignment.

(continued on next page)

fig. 1

TREE POSE (cont.)

4. Inhale to bring the palms of the hands back to the heart center (fig. 2). Exhale to gently lower the leg to the ground with control. Practice the pose on the opposite side.

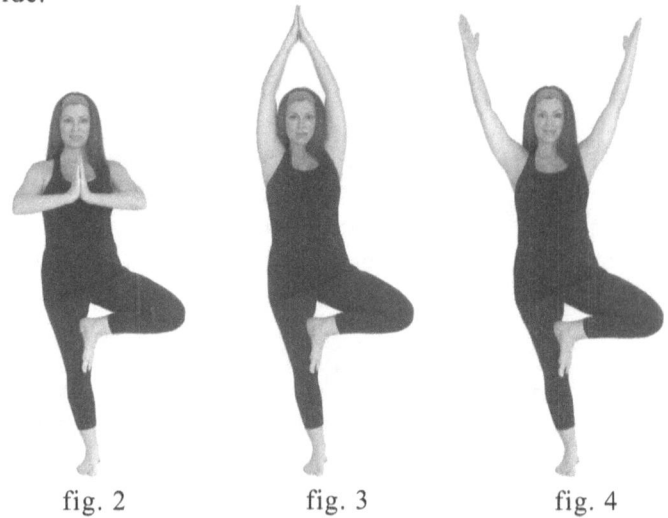

fig. 2   fig. 3   fig. 4

STRADDLE SPLITS

Benefits: This posture is a wonderful Hip opener. It works on loosening and opening the pelvic area, keeping the lower back limber and strengthening the legs to give an easier labor.

1. Begin by stepping out wide onto the mat with the hands resting on the hips (fig. 1, next page). The feet should be slightly pigeon- toed so that the outside edges of the feet stay parallel.

(continued on next page)

STRADDLE SPLITS (cont.)

2. Inhale to lengthen through the torso and as you exhale, hinge from your hips (fig. 2) and bring the hands to the floor beneath the shoulders or onto blocks if you have them (fig. 3).

3. Try bringing the body weight forward into the balls of the feet to keep the hips in the same plane as the ankles and knees. Relax the neck as the crown of the head aims downward toward the ground. Lengthen through the spine and engage the thigh muscles and draw them upwards. Stay here for a few breaths, lengthening the spine and hamstrings on the inhales and deepening the forward bend on the exhales. If you'd like a further stretch, open the feet wider.

4. To come out of this pose, bring the hands onto the hips while keeping the back flat slowly lift the body to a standing position (fig. 2, then fig. 1). Repeat 3 times.

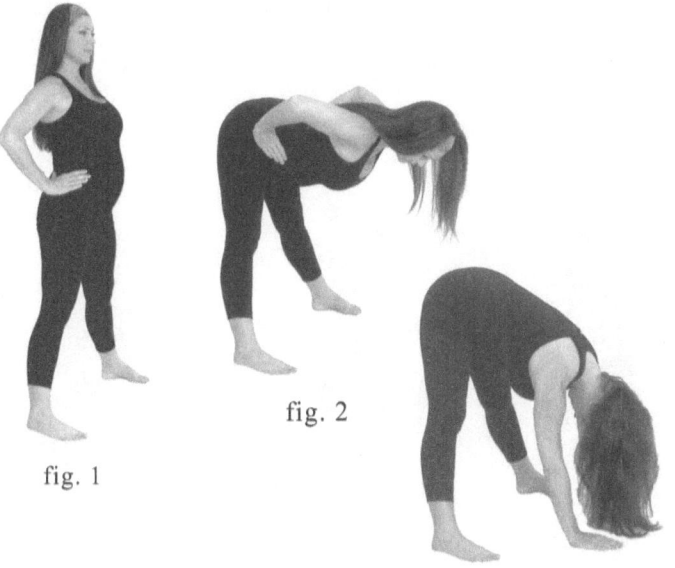

fig. 2

fig. 1

fig. 3

SQUAT AND RISE POSE

Benefits: This posture is recommended daily throughout your pregnancy. Squatting helps to relax and open the pelvis and strengthen the upper legs. Squats will assist in preparation for your delivery.

1. Separate the feet at least hip width apart or wider with the feet flat on the floor. Interlace the fingers in front of you and let the arms and hands hang loosely in front of you (fig. 1). For this pose, keep the heels on the floor throughout. But if they do not reach, place a rolled up blanket or towel beneath them.

2. Inhale to prepare and as you exhale gently bend the knees and lower the body ¼ of the way down while focusing on pulling the tailbone downward and engaging the pelvic floor muscles (fig. 2).

3. Inhale to extend upwards again and exhale gently bending the knees a little further about ½ the way down (fig. 3). Feel the energy of pressing down mimicking the flow of energy when birthing.

(continued next page)

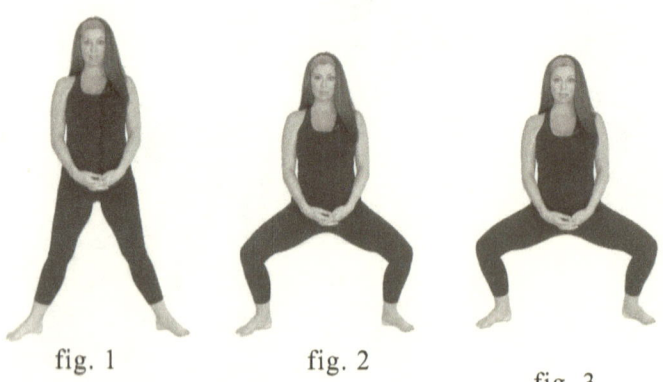

fig. 1   fig. 2

fig. 3

SQUAT AND RISE POSE (cont.)

4. Inhale and straighten the legs to extend upwards and exhale to sit ¾ of the way down. Inhale to stand and without resting, exhale as you squat all the way down to the ground (figs. 4 & 5).

5. Return to a standing posture. Repeat this sequence working up to ten times.

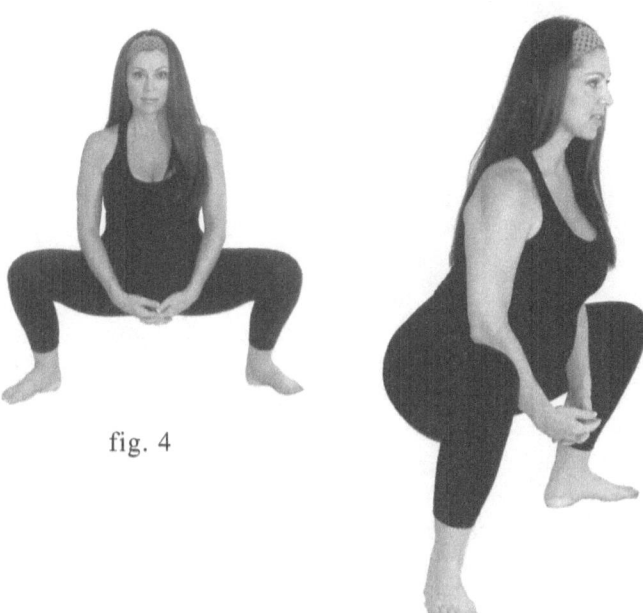

fig. 4

fig. 5

FLOOR EXERCISES

CAT/COW POSE

Benefits: Cat/Cow pose is a wonderful exercise through-out your pregnancy to relieve discomfort from carrying your baby all day. The fluid movements synchronized with breath will stretch your spine, relieve back pain, strengthen your arms and in the final stages of preg-nancy, help get your baby into optimal position for childbirth.

1. Come to a kneeling position with the knees slightly apart beneath the hips and hands beneath the shoulders. Place the palms of the hands flat on the floor and finger-tips spread open wide and relax the tops of the feet onto the floor (fig. 1).

2. Inhale and raise the head and look upwards while aiming the tailbone toward the ceiling and dipping the middle back downwards slightly (fig. 2). Feel the stretch across the chest and the heart center open.

3. Exhale and round the back by tucking the tailbone down to the ground and tucking the chin in toward the chest. Round your spine slowly all the way to the shoul-ders and head (fig. 3).

4. Continue to move with the breath back and forth into both positions coordinating the breath and movement. Repeat 5 times.

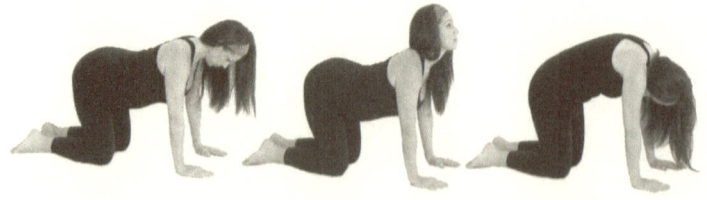

fig. 1   fig. 2   fig. 3

SPINAL BALANCING WITH LEG LIFTS

Benefits: This exercise helps to strengthen and lengthen your back and spinal muscles. It also helps with core control and balance. Spinal Balancing will also allow increased focus and concentration.

1. Come to a kneeling position with the knees slightly apart beneath the hips and hands beneath the shoulders. Place the palms of the hands flat on the floor and finger-tips spread open wide and relax the tops of the feet onto the floor (fig. 1).

2. Inhale to extend the right leg back behind you and exhale to extend the left arm out in front of you (fig. 2). Feel the length of your spine and feel the strength of your core. Reach through your fingertips and reach through your toes.

3. Inhale as you slowly lower the right leg downward towards the ground (fig. 3) and exhale as you lift the leg back up. Repeat this movement 5 times.

4. Gently release the leg down to the ground while placing the knee on the floor (fig. 1) and lower your arm and hand as well. Repeat on the opposite side.

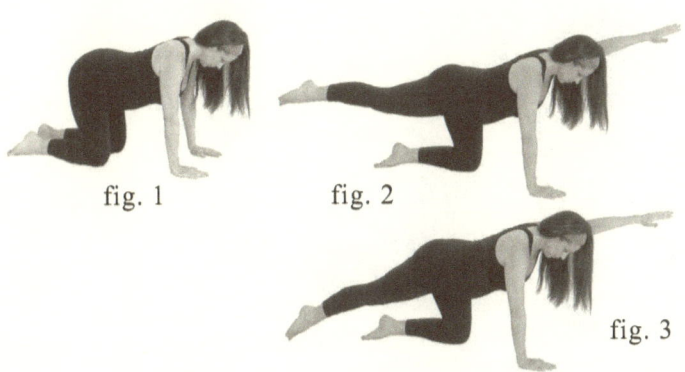

fig. 1   fig. 2

fig. 3

PELVIC CIRCLES

Benefits: Pelvic Circles stretch and loosen up the hips and pelvis. It is great to relieve back pain from carrying your baby all day. This exercise also builds core strength and spinal flexibility.

1. Come to a kneeling position with the knees slightly apart beneath the hips and hands about 12 inches forward in front of the shoulders (fig. 1). The palms of the hands lie flat on the floor and fingertips spread open wide. Relax the tops of the feet onto the floor.

2. Imagine the pelvis as a clock. Begin to move the hips to the 9 o'clock position, then to the 6 o'clock position, over to the 3 o'clock position and then forward to the 12 o'clock position (figs. 2 thru 5).

3. Coordinate the breath with the movement. Repeat 3 to 5 times and switch directions.

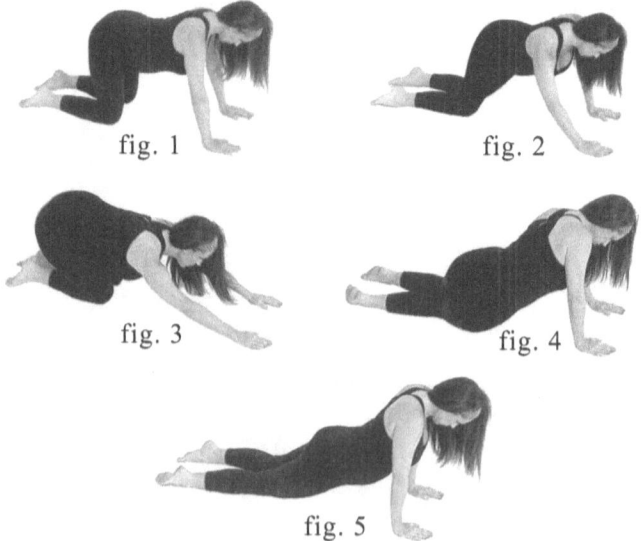

fig. 1

fig. 2

fig. 3

fig. 4

fig. 5

CHILD'S POSE

Benefits: This posture is a wonderfully relaxing pose during pregnancy. This is a resting and restorative pose. Child's Pose is soothing to the mind, body and emotions. Physically, this posture helps to relieve lower back pain as well as hip and thigh pain. It also encourages blood flow to the kidneys and adrenal glands. Mentally, this pose helps to relieve fatigue and stress by slowing down the body and putting you more in touch with your breath.

1. Begin by sitting with the hips on the heels. Press downward with the hips while lengthening upward through the spine.

2. Exhale and slightly engage the core as you hinge forward from the hips bringing the torso over the thighs (fig. 1). Bring the forehead toward the floor and extend the arms forward.

3. Focus on deep slow rhythmic breaths.

*HINT
If there is any discomfort in the neck or shoulders while the arms are extended forward, extend the arms along the sides of the body. If the hips do not reach the heels or if there is knee pain, place a cushion between the buttocks and heels. You may also open the knees out wider for more comfort. If the forehead does not reach the floor place a small towel or blanket under the forehead or rest the forehead on top of the fists. If you have sensitivity in the ankles possibly due to swelling then place a folded towel or blanket under the ankles.

fig. 1

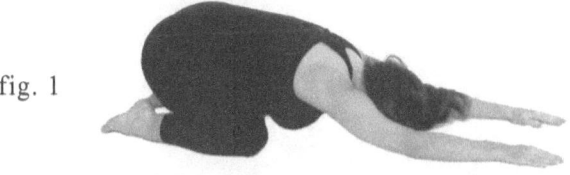

LUNGE

Benefits: This exercise will build strength and endurance in the entire body. Lunges help to strengthen the legs, open the hips, and help you to feel more balanced. Lunges will also teach physical and mental strength, both of which are important during child birth.

1. Begin on all fours (fig. 1). Step the right foot forward between the hands with the knee over the ankle (fig. 2). Stretch the left leg back, keep the left knee on the ground and sink the pelvis toward the ground.

2. To move deeper into this Lunge, rest both hands onto the forward knee and press down through the pelvis, enjoying the stretch on the front of that leg (fig. 3). Lift up through the crown of the head and open the chest, arching the back ever so slightly. To go even deeper now, straighten the left leg raising the knee off of the ground and by curling the toes forward.

(continued on next page)

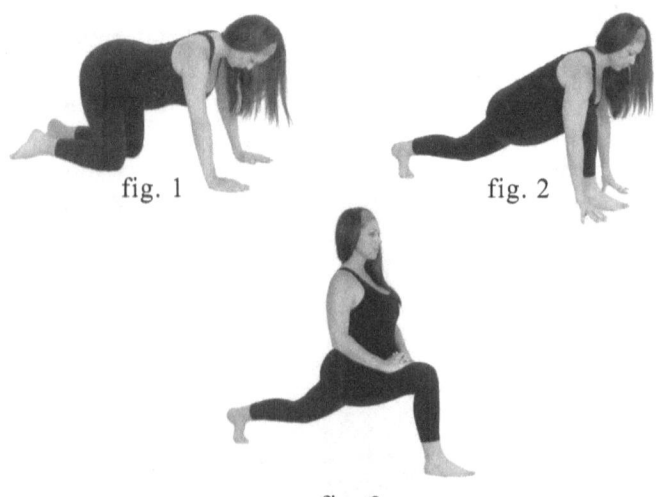

fig. 1

fig. 2

fig. 3

LUNGE (cont.)

3. To challenge yourself further, inhale the arms up overhead and reach to the ceiling extending through the fingertips (fig. 4). Pull the tailbone downward, and open the chest and heart by arching the back slightly. Inhale deeply and as you exhale gently lower the hands to your thigh and back down to the floor. Release the back leg as well. Step the left foot back and prepare to Lunge on the opposite side. Repeat on opposite side and repeat 3 times on each side.

fig. 4

STRIKING COBRA POSE

Benefits: Striking Cobra Pose allows for great flexibility to the spine, tones the spinal muscles and relieves back pain. This pose also strengthens the shoulders, opens the chest and gives a nice stretch in the abdominals.

1. From all fours extend the hands slightly out in front of the shoulders (fig. 1). Inhale and slowly lower the hips towards the floor, taking the weight of the body into the arms and tilting the head upwards toward the ceiling (fig. 2). Exhale to open the heart and the chest pressing your shoulder blades down and enjoy this wonderful stretch in the front of the body.

2. Slowly return to the all fours position. Repeat 3 times.

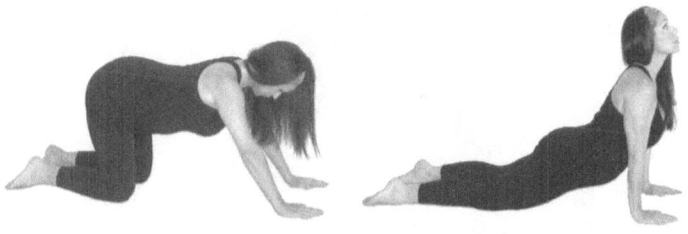

fig. 1   fig. 2

DOWNWARD FACING DOG POSE

Benefits: This pose gives the whole posterior body a stretch, from the back of the legs through the entire spine to the head.

1. From all fours and with the fingertips spread wide, inhale and curl the toes forward with the heels raised up (fig. 1).

2. Exhale to straighten the legs and raise the hips into the air. Relax the head in line with the level of the arms (fig. 2). Press the heels into the ground and shift the chest towards the knees (fig. 3). Straighten the back. Feel the length of the spine stretching and elongating. Enjoy this wonderful full body stretch.

3. To release the posture come down to the starting position on the hands and knees. Repeat 3 times.

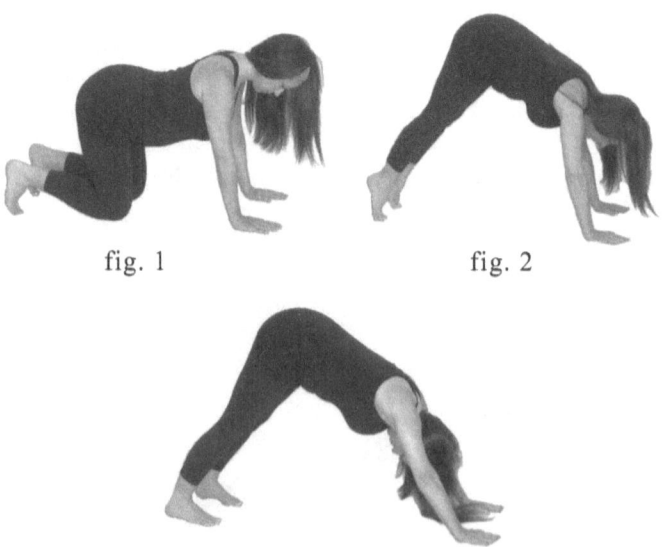

fig. 1   fig. 2

fig. 3

PLANK POSE

Benefits: Plank Pose strengthens the abs, paraspinals and shoulders. This pose helps to keep the core strong which helps with back pain and discomfort during pregnancy.

1. From an all fours position spread the fingertips wide (fig. 1). Inhale to curl the toes forward and exhale to straighten the legs and raise the hips into the air (fig. 2). Inhale and draw the torso forward until the shoulders are over the wrists and the whole body is in one straight line (fig. 3). Tuck the tailbone and engage the abdominals.

2. Exhale while pressing the forearms and hands firmly down. Do not let the chest sink. Press back through the heels. Keep the neck in alignment with the spine. Feel the strength of the core. Hold the position for a few breaths.

3. To release, bend the knees and return to an all fours position.

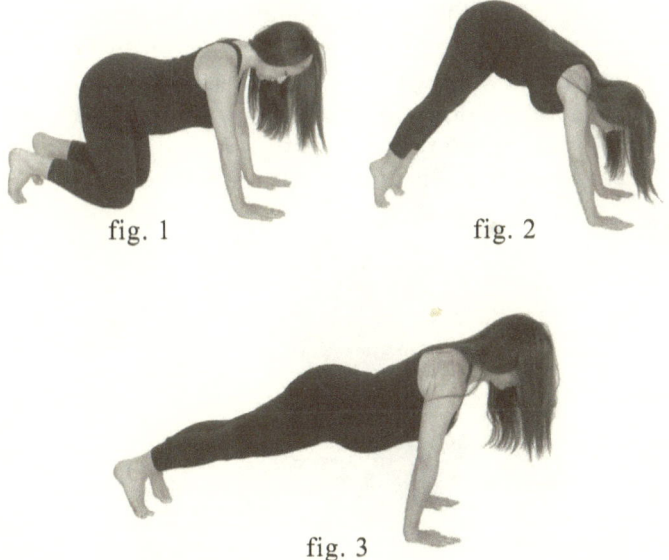

fig. 1   fig. 2

fig. 3

SEATED POSES

BUTTERFLY STRETCH WITH A STRAP

Benefits: This pose is extremely beneficial during pregnancy as it opens the whole pelvic area, stretching your hips, inner thighs and lower back muscles. All of these muscles play a major role in preparation for child-birth.

1. Come to a comfortable seated position bringing the soles of the feet together in front of the body with the knees apart. Loop the strap around the toes and pull the heels in close (fig. 1).

2. Straighten up through your spine while reaching the crown of your head toward the ceiling. Lift your chest and sternum upward and relax your shoulder blades downward.

3. Begin using the leg muscles and raising and lowering both knees upward toward the shoulders and then actively pressing them downward towards the ground. Just breathe freely and relax through the inner thighs. Allow the legs to bounce up and down as you release tension. Gradually go a bit faster relaxing the inner thighs. Repeat for up to 20 repetitions then relax and repeat 2 more times.

fig. 1

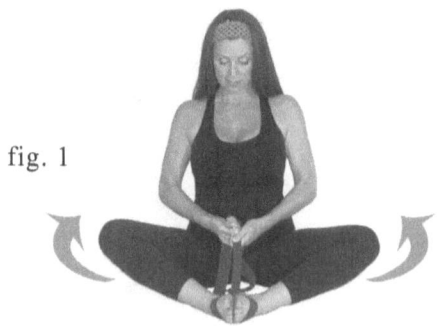

SEATED SPINAL TWIST

Benefits: This pose benefits the internal organs by improving digestion and the processing of the liver and kidneys. It helps to relieve backaches and generate more mobility in the spine and hips.This pose releases tension, generates a sense of well-being, and rejuvenates the entire body and mind.

1. Begin in a seated position with the spine erect and the legs extended (fig. 1). Bend the right knee in placing the foot onto the floor. Bring the left hand onto the right knee and right hand behind the back close to the sacrum. Sit up tall pressing the shoulder blades downward.

2. Inhale and as you exhale slowly begin to twist the body first at the navel, then at the rib cage and then at the shoulders (fig. 2). Gaze over the right shoulder. Press through the crown of the head and lengthen up through the spine. Hold the twist for several breaths moving deeper and relaxing more fully with each breath.

3. Exhale to gently untwist and return the body to the starting position. Repeat on the opposite side.

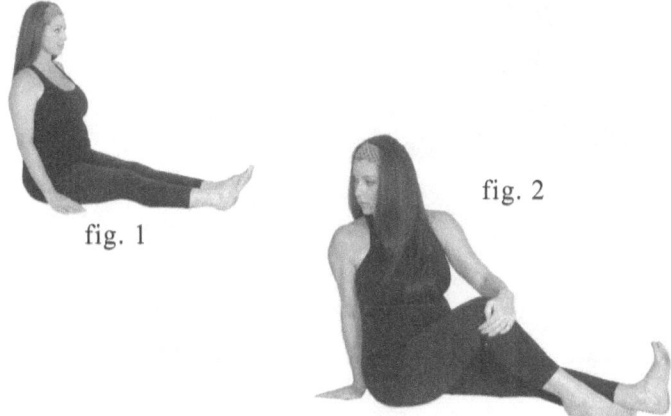

fig. 1

fig. 2

CHURNING THE MILL

Benefits: This excellent yoga posture massages and strengthens abdominal muscles and the organs of the pelvis, preparing them for pregnancy.

1. Begin in a seated position with the legs wide, feet far apart, and interlock the fingers forward (fig. 1). Rotate the body over toward the right foot (fig. 2). Lean fully forward towards the right foot.

2. Rotate the body at the waist circling the hands across to the left foot and then lean backwards circling the hands over the groin from left to the right and then back to the right foot again. Make strong pushing and pulling movements as if stirring a pot of soup as you circle the body (figs. 2 thru 4).

3. Match the breath to the movement repeating for 10 circles and switch directions of the circle.

*HINT
 If you are experiencing any back problems do not over-stretch in the forward bend.

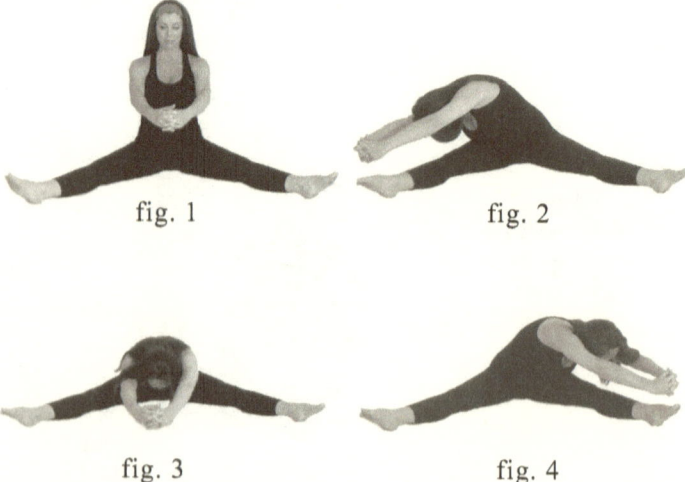

fig. 1   fig. 2

fig. 3   fig. 4

ROLL DOWNS

Benefits: Roll Downs will really put you in touch with your abdominals. They will also give you a wonderful hamstring and spine stretch. I recommend the full version of Roll Downs with extended legs only during your first trimester and the modified version with bent knees for your second trimester.

1. Begin in a seated upright position with the legs extended (first trimester) or with feet slightly out in front of the body, feet flat onto the mat (second trimester) (fig 1). Hold onto the back of the thighs or reach the arms out in front of the shoulders.

2. Inhale and as you exhale draw the navel in toward the spine and slowly begin to roll down through the spine one bone at a time. Reach the arms back and behind the head (fig. 2).

3. Inhale as you bring the arms straight up towards the ceiling and exhale to reach upwards through the fingertips lifting the head neck and shoulders off of the ground. Stretch forward toward the toes while extending your legs straight (fig. 3).

(continued on next page)

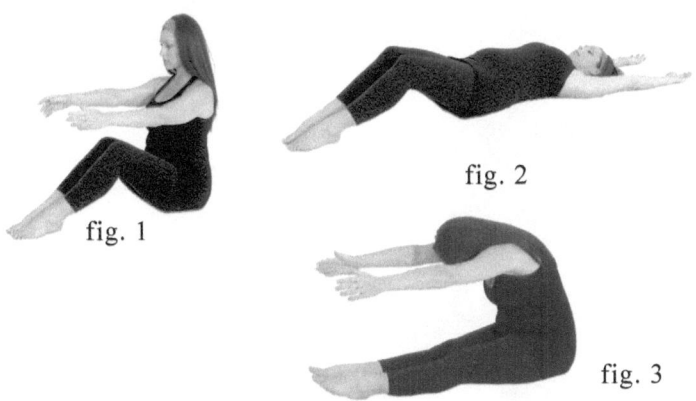

fig. 1

fig. 2

fig. 3

ROLL DOWNS (cont.)

4.Hold and feel the stretch from the toes all the way up the back of the legs and up the spine to the crown of the head. Bend the knees again by planting the feet onto the floor and exhale as you gently roll down through the spine. Easily and gently place one bone down at a time. Repeat 5 times.

LYING ON THE BACK EXERCISES/POSES

SINGLE ALTERNATE LEG LOWERS

Benefits: This exercise helps to develop strength and relaxation of the legs, as well as the abdominals.

1. Lie on the back while relaxing the arms beside the body. Keep the body in a neutral spinal alignment. Bend both knees in toward the chest (fig. 1) and then extend the legs upward towards the ceiling (fig. 2). Reach long from the hip sockets all the way up to the toes.

2. Inhale to slowly lower the right leg toward the floor and exhale to slowly lift (fig. 3 & 4). Inhale to lower the left leg and exhale to slowly lift. Keep the abdominals contracted throughout by drawing the navel in toward the spine.

3. Continue to alternate leg lowers keeping the tailbone on the ground. Try to allow only the legs to move keeping the entire torso steady and strong. Repeat 10 times with each leg.

4. To release, gently bend both knees and slowly lower the legs to the ground. Extend your legs straight and shake them out.

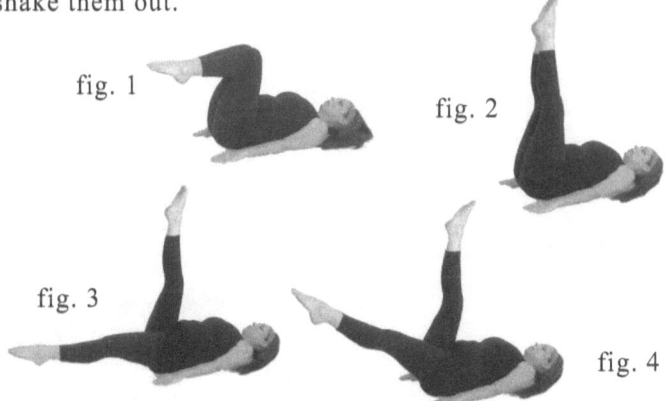

fig. 1

fig. 2

fig. 3

fig. 4

DOUBLE LEG LOWERS

Benefits: In pregnancy, the legs bear the majority
of weight gained by the growing abdomen. Double Leg
Lowers will develop strength in your legs.

1. Lie on the back while relaxing the arms beside the
body. Keep the body in a neutral spinal alignment. Bend
both knees in toward the chest (fig. 1) and then extend the
legs upward towards the ceiling (fig. 2). Reach long from
the hip sockets all the way up to the toes.

2. Inhale to gently lower both legs together as far as you
can without bending the knees (fig. 3). When you have
lowered as far as possible, bend the knees and then slowly
exhale to lift them back up. Keep the abdominal muscles
engaged and match your breath to a smooth controlled
movement.

3. To release, gently bend both knees and slowly lower
the legs to the ground. Extend your legs straight and
shake them out. Repeat 5 times.

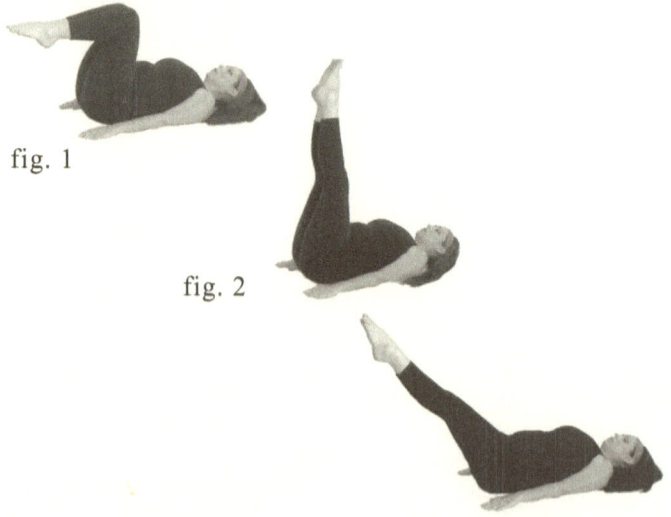

fig. 1

fig. 2

fig. 3

WIDE LEGGED V'S

Benefits: Wide Legged V's not only strengthen your legs but also allow for a wonderful inner thigh opening and hamstring stretch.

1. Bend the knees into the chest and extend the legs straight up towards the ceiling. Engage the abdominal muscles and keep the spine in a neutral alignment. Open the arms out wide in alignment with the shoulders, palms pressing downward. Flex the feet and press through the heels (fig. 1).

2. Inhale as you open the legs in a wide V (figs. 2 & 3). Hold this and feel the stretch. Exhale as you engage the inner thigh muscles and bring the legs back together. Move at your own pace, coordinating the breath with the flow of the body. Draw the navel deep into the spine as you bring the legs together. Enjoy the freedom this stretch brings and breathe through it deeply. Open up and release the inner thigh muscles. Repeat 10 times.

3. To release bend the knees and gently lower the legs to the floor and extend the legs straight out.

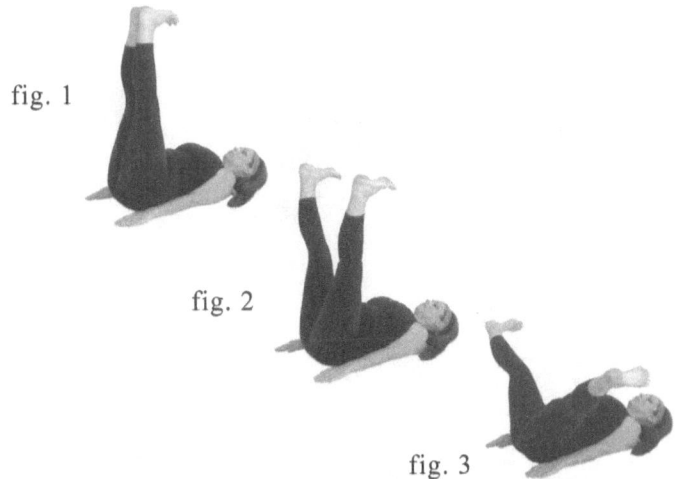

fig. 1

fig. 2

fig. 3

SINGLE LEG CIRCLES

Benefits: This exercise helps to loosen your hips, strengthen your legs and stretch your hamstrings. Single Leg Circles also strengthen the abdominal muscles.

1. Begin lying flat on the back with the arms by your sides. Bend the right knee into the chest and then extend the right leg up towards the ceiling. Keep the knee aligned with the hip (fig. 1).

2. Without moving the hips, inhale and cross the right leg over the body swinging it past the left leg circling around and down and then exhale to reach back up toward the ceiling (figs. 2 thru 4). Keep the leg within the frame of the shoulders.

3. Focus on matching the breath to the movement. Breathe slowly and deeply and relax throughout releasing tension in the hip. Repeat 4 more times. Reverse the direction of the circle and repeat 5 times.

4. Switch to the opposite leg. Circle 5 times in each direction.

fig. 1

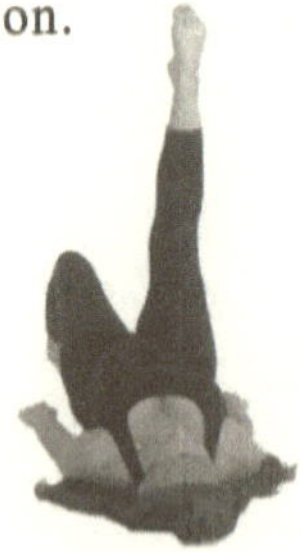

fig. 2

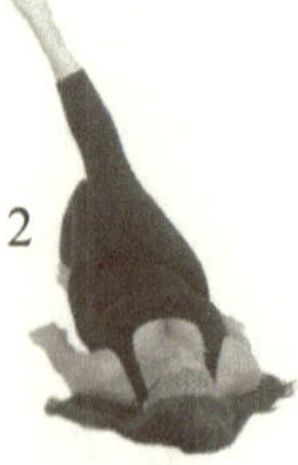

fig. 3

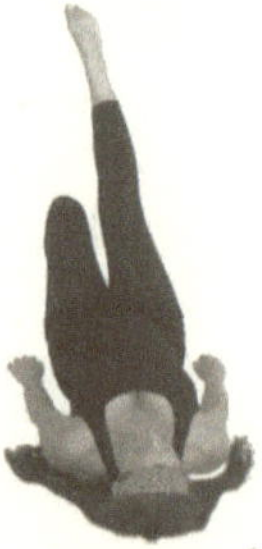

fig. 4

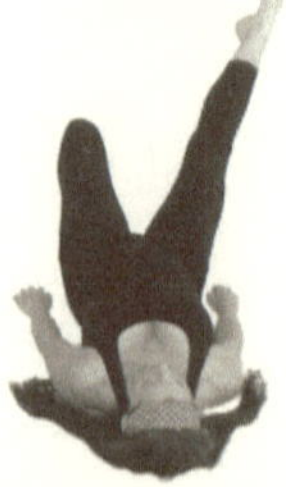

SHOULDER POSE

Benefits: Shoulder Pose is an energizing modified back-bend. It enables flexibility of the spine, relieves lower back pain, develops strength in the legs and uterus. It also encourages deep breathing.

1. Lie on the back with both knees bent and the soles of the feet flat on the floor. Place the heels close into the buttocks. The feet and knees are hip width apart. Relax the hands beside the hips (fig. 1).

2. Inhale slowly and gently push the hips up into the air as far as is comfortable for you (figs. 2 & 3). Hold for a few moments. Press the feet downward into the floor and the hips upward toward the ceiling.

3. Exhale to slowly lower the body. Repeat 5 times.

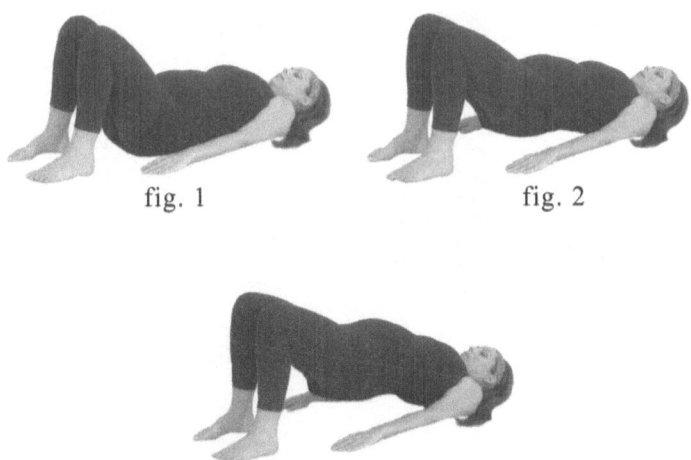

fig. 1   fig. 2

fig. 3

SINGLE STRAIGHT LEG STRETCH

Benefits: This exercise offers a wonderful hamstring stretch. It increases overall flexibility in your legs. Your core muscles will also feel a great workout.

1. Bring the right leg straight up towards the ceiling and point the toes of the right foot. Extend your left leg out in front of you, pointing the toes. Inhale and grab a hold of the back of the right calf or thigh (fig. 1).

2. Tuck the chin in towards the chest while lifting the head neck and shoulders off of the ground. Press the shoulder blades down and away from the ears. Draw the navel in towards the spine.

3. Exhale and draw the right calf (or thigh) in closer towards the chest and pulse the leg for 2 times pulling it gently toward you.

4. And like scissors, switch legs bringing the left leg towards you and pulsing the left leg twice (fig. 2).The movements are quick. Repeat 10 times.

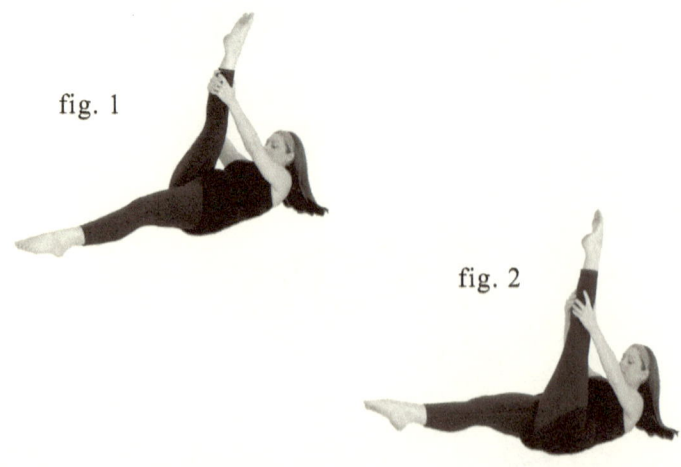

fig. 1

fig. 2

HAPPY BABY POSE

Benefits: This is a fun pose during pregnancy. It gently stretches the inner groins and the back spine. Happy baby pose also helps to calm the brain and relieves stress and fatigue.

1. Lie on the back and bend the knees into the chest (fig. 1). Open the knees bringing them towards the armpits. Grip the outsides of the feet with the hands (fig. 2). Align the ankles over the knees so that the shins are perpendicular to the floor. Flex the feet.

2. Gently push the feet up into the hands as you pull the hands down to create a resistance. Coax the thighs in toward the torso and downward toward the floor as you lengthen the spine and release the tail bone toward the ground. Inhale deeply into your back spine and exhale completely to move deeper into this inner groin and back stretch (fig. 3). Enjoy the release of the tailbone further and further toward the ground.

3. Hold the pose steadily for 30 seconds to one minute.

4. To come out of the pose slowly release the hands and bring the legs together. Lower the feet back to the ground and extend your legs straight out.

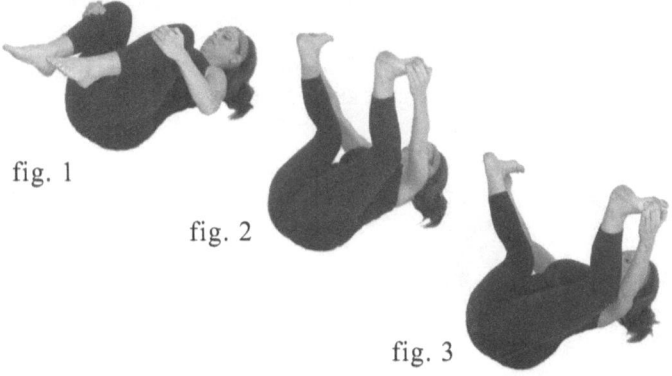

fig. 1

fig. 2

fig. 3

BODY LENGTHENING

Benefits: This final posture helps to release and let go of any remaining tensions within. Body Lengthening allows every muscle in the body to be free to melt and meld together as one while helping to prepare you for meditation.

1. Lie on the back and open the legs out wide into a V and extend your arms overhead and open into a wide V as well. Stretch your whole entire body long and relax (fig. 1, next page).

2. Inhale and lift the right leg up off of the floor about 2-3 inches, engage the thigh muscle, point the toes and reach the right leg as long as you can and stretch from the hip all the way to the tips of the toes. Exhale and relax the leg back to the ground.

3. Inhale and lift the left leg up off of the floor about 2-3 inches, engage the thigh muscle, point the toes and reach the left leg as long as you can and stretch from the hip all the way to the tips of the toes. Exhale and relax the leg back to the ground.

4. Inhale and lift the right arm off of the floor 2-3 inches and reach your right arm as long as you can. Reach through the fingers to the fingertips and stretch. Tighten up all of the muscles in your arm. Make a fist. Squeeze the hand and then open the hand and reach the fingertips as long as you can. Exhale and relax the right arm to the ground.

(continued next page)

BODY LENGTHENING (cont.)

5. Inhale and lift the left arm off of the floor 2-3 inches and reach the left arm as long as you can. Reach through the fingers to the fingertips and stretch. Tighten up all of the muscles in the arm. Make a fist. Squeeze the hand and then open the hand and reach the fingertips as long as you can. Exhale and relax the left arm to the ground.

6. Inhale and lift the entire body, both legs and arms and reach in both directions. Feel the stretch in the entire body. Squeeze every muscle tight in the body. Feel the elongation of every muscle. Reach and lengthen the whole body as long as possible and just RELAX. Release every muscle in the body and REST.

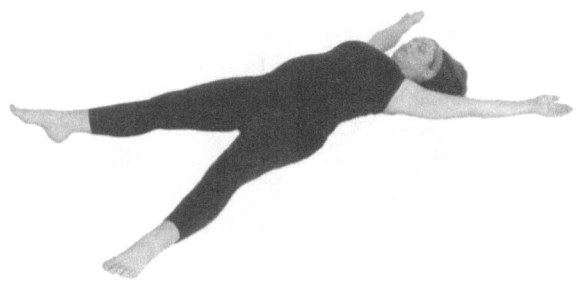

fig. 1

Third Trimester Essentials

Note: It is extremely important as you enter your Third Trimester that you consult with your physician on a regular basis as to the amount and type of exercising you should be doing. As always, use common sense and listen to your body!

Some of the exercises from the First and Second Trimester that **should not** be done in your Third Trimester are: **Cobra, Plank, Cow Pose, Roll Downs and Double Leg Lowers.**

The following exercises can be done in the Third Trimester almost exactly as in the First and Second. Any slight differences when performing these exercises are noted.

Mountain Pose - NOTE: Be sure to tuck the tailbone slightly to prevent an arch in the lower back. This will help to prevent lower back pain. If lifting onto the toes is not possible for you at this time, perform the posture with the feet flat on the ground.

Chest Expansion - NOTE: Like all standing poses, be mindful of straight alignment and of not arching through the back. To allow less of a stretch through the chest, open the hands out wider on the strap and do not extend as far back behind the shoulders.

Yoga Mudra - NOTE: For more comfort, step the feet out wider than hip width. If there is tension in the chest, open the hands out wider onto the strap.

Arm Circles - NOTE: As you raise the arms overhead, avoid arching the back slightly as you did in the First and Second Trimester. Keep the spine long and the tailbone aiming toward the floor.

(continued next page)

Third Trimester Essentials (cont.)

Pelvic Circles - No changes, except you may wish to use a pillow under your knees.
Happy Baby Pose - NOTE: Place both hands onto the knees rather than the soles of the feet. Rock your pelvis from side to side to soothe the lower back. Hold this pose for 30 seconds to 1 minute only.

The following pages contain those exercises that will need to be adapted with the addition of a chair, pillow or the position that you use when performing the exercise.
   Please continue your exercising as long as it is physician approved. It won't be long now until you'll be bringing a new life into the world!

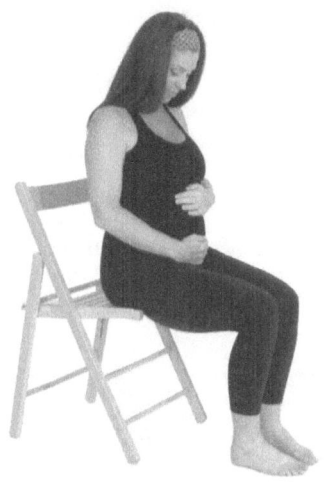

CHAIR POSES

SQUATS

1. Separate the feet wider than hip width apart. Feet flat on the floor. Stand behind a chair and hold lightly to assist with balance (fig. 1).

2. Inhale to prepare and as you exhale gently bend the knees and lower the body ¼ of the way down while focusing on pulling the tailbone downward and engaging the pelvic floor muscles (fig. 2).

3. Inhale to extend upwards again and exhale gently bending the knees a little further about ½ the way down. Feel the energy of pressing down, mimicking the flow of energy when birthing (fig. 3).

4. Inhale and straighten the legs to extend upwards and exhale to sit all the way down to the ground in a full squat (fig. 4).

5. Return to a standing posture. Repeat this sequence, working up to ten times.
*HINT - Open the knees wider for more comfort if necessary. If the heels do not reach the floor, place a rolled up towel or blanket beneath them.

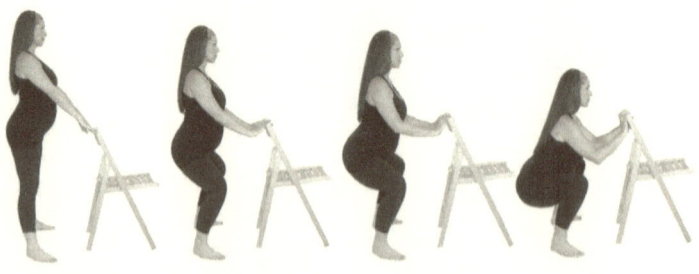

fig. 1   fig. 2   fig. 3   fig. 4

LUNGE

1. Stand behind a chair with feet hip width apart (fig. 1).
Reach the arms forward to hold onto chair for balance.

2. Inhale and stretch the right leg back, placing the right
ball of the foot onto the floor. Bend the right knee to
lower the body downward into a Lunge. Step back far
enough so that the end result is that of the left knee being
directly over the left ankle (fig. 2).

3. Exhale to return to the starting position. Repeat 5
times and switch legs.

*HINT
Breathe slowly and deeply throughout. Do not hold the
breath.

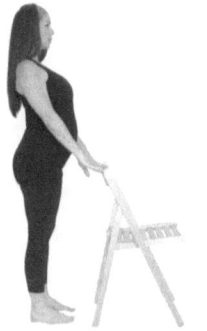   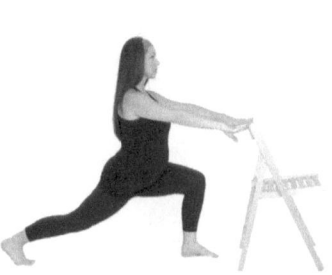

fig. 1   fig. 2

PILATES ONE FOOT BALANCE

1. Stand behind or beside a chair with the feet hip width apart. Draw the tailbone slightly downward and engage the core. Begin by shifting all of the weight to the right foot. Feel all four corners of the right foot pressing into the ground. Lift the knee cap upward toward the hip by engaging the right thigh muscle. Feel a strong line of energy from the heel up to your hip.

2. Raise the right arm out to the side of the body in alignment with the shoulder with the palm pressing downward. Hold onto the chair with the left hand.

3. Inhale the right leg up bringing the knee in alignment with the hip (fig. 1). Inhale to lower the leg touching the big toe to the ground and exhale as you engage in the pelvic floor to lift the leg back up. Repeat 5 times.

4. Extend the leg straight (fig. 2) and then inhale to lower the straight leg toward the ground and exhale to lift the leg. Repeat 5 times. Switch legs.

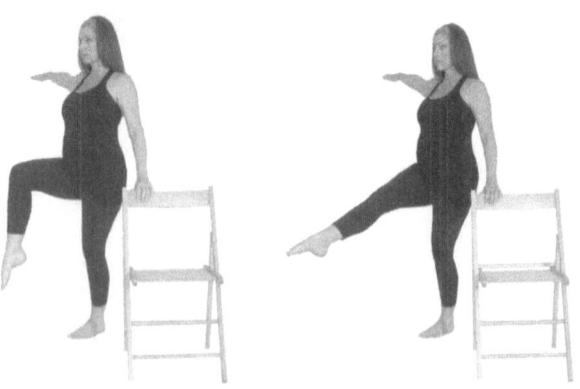

fig. 1   fig. 2

TREE POSE

1. Stand behind or beside a chair with the feet hip width apart, tailbone aiming downward and relax the arms by your sides. Press evenly through the feet engaging the thigh muscles. Lift the pelvic floor muscles and engage the core. Focus at a point about 45 degrees below eye level in front of you. Shift all of the weight to the right foot and feel a strong line of energy from the heel up to your hip. Do not lock the knee.

2. Hold onto the chair with the right hand. Inhale and place the sole of the left foot either over the opposite ankle, higher up the leg pressing into the calf or against the inner thigh of the right leg (fig. 1). Exhale to relax. Press down through the right foot and reach the crown of the head up toward the ceiling.

3. Inhale the left arm overhead and reach the fingertips toward the ceiling (fig. 2). Lift out of the waist, feeling this wonderful stretch in your abdomen. Hold for a few breaths. Focus on keeping the hips square and maintaining a neutral spinal alignment.

4. Inhale to lower the arm by the side. Exhale to gently lower the leg to the ground with control. Practice the pose on the opposite side.

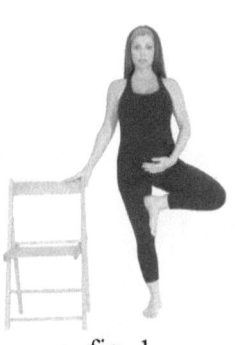

fig. 1

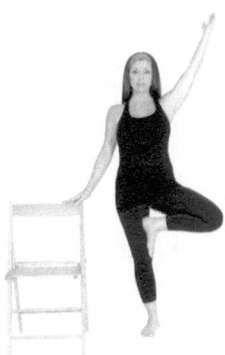

fig. 2

STRADDLE SPLITS

1. Place a chair out in front of you. Step out wide onto the mat with the hands resting on the hips. The feet should be slightly pigeon-toed so that the outside edges of the feet stay parallel (fig. 1).

2. Inhale to lengthen through the torso and as you exhale, hinge from your hips and bring the hands onto the chair in front of you (fig. 2).

3. Try bringing the body weight forward into the balls of the feet to keep the hips in the same plane as the ankles and knees. Relax the neck as the crown of the head aims downward. Lengthen through the spine and engage the thigh muscles and draw them upwards. To move deeper into the pose bring the forearms onto the chair and hold for a few breaths. If possible, bring the palms of the hands onto the ground (fig. 3).

4. To come out of this pose, bring the hands onto the chair or onto the hips. Keep the back flat and slowly lift the body to a standing position. Repeat 3 times.

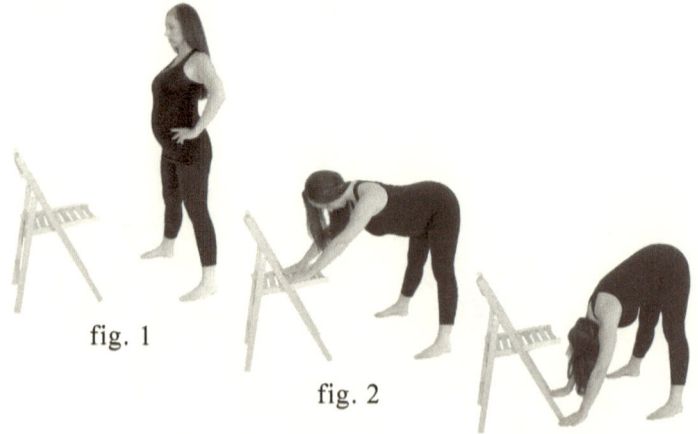

fig. 1

fig. 2

fig. 3

FLOOR EXERCISES

CAT POSE

1. Come to a kneeling position with the knees slightly apart resting on a pillow beneath the hips and hands beneath the shoulders. Place the palms of the hands flat on the floor and fingertips spread open wide and relax the tops of the feet onto the floor (fig. 1).

2. Inhale as you look straight out in front of you while maintaining a flat back.

3. Exhale as you round the back while tucking the chin towards the chest and the tailbone toward the ground (fig. 2).

4. Repeat 5 times focusing on the pelvic floor contraction on the exhale.

*HINT
Avoid arching the back while in the straight position as this can cause discomfort.

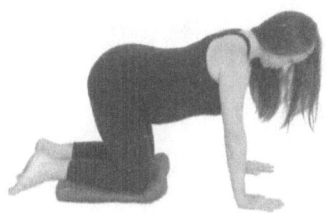

fig. 1

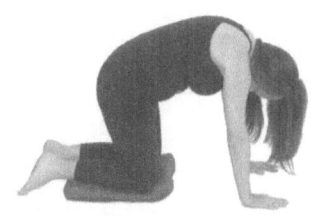

fig. 2

SPINAL BALANCING

1. Come to a kneeling position with the knees slightly apart beneath the hips resting onto a pillow and hands beneath the shoulders. Place the palms of the hands flat on the floor and fingertips spread open wide and relax the tops of the feet onto the floor (fig. 1).

2. Inhale to extend the right arm out in front of you. Feel the length of your spine and feel the strength of your core. Reach through your fingertips while focusing on your balance (fig. 2).

3. Exhale to release the hand back to the floor. Switch to the opposite arm. Repeat this movement 5 times.
*HINT
Keep the spine long and avoid arching the lower back.

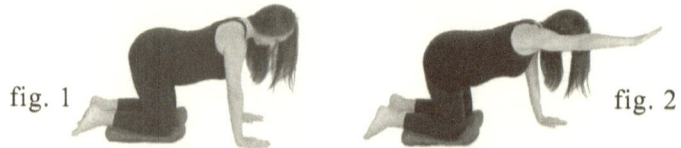

fig. 1   fig. 2

LEG LIFTS   fig. 3

1. Same start as above.

2. Inhale to extend the right leg
back behind you and exhale to hold the position (fig.3).

3. Inhale to lower the right leg downward toward the floor and exhale to lift.

4. Repeat 5 times and then switch to the opposite leg.
If you experience any lower back discomfort, discontinue the exercise.

PELVIC CIRCLES

NOTE: Pelvic Circles will be performed exactly as during the First and Second Trimesters (page 32), with the exception of a pillow under the knees (if needed) for added comfort as shown below.

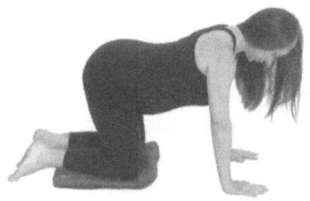

CHILD'S POSE

NOTE: Child's Pose will be performed exactly as during the First and Second Trimesters (page 33), with the exception of a pillow under the knees (if needed) for added comfort as shown below. Also, if your hips do not comfortably reach your heels, use a second pillow as shown below.

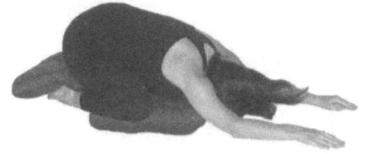

SEATED POSES

HALF BUTTERFLY STRETCH

1. Begin seated onto a pillow allowing a slightly forward tilt of the pelvis. Bend the right leg and place the right foot beside and as close to the right inner thigh as is possible (fig. 1).

2. Begin using the leg muscle and raising and lowering the right knee upward toward the shoulder and then actively pressing downward towards the ground. Allow the leg to bounce up and down as you release tension. Gradually go a bit faster, relaxing the inner thigh. Repeat for up to 10 repetitions.

3. Release the foot and shake out the leg. Switch to the opposite leg.

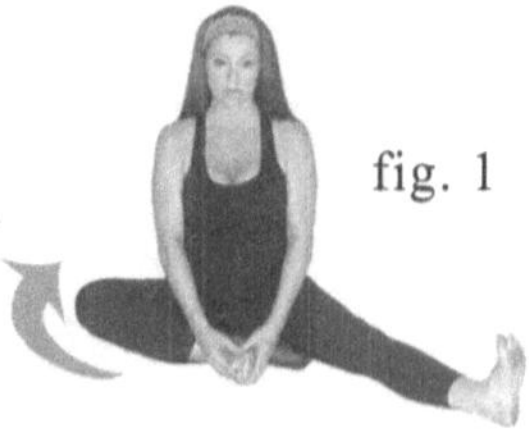

fig. 1

SIDE BEND STRETCH

1. Begin in a comfortable seated position onto a pillow. Place both legs to the left side of the body.

2. Place the left arm on to the floor. Inhale to extend the right arm up towards the ceiling and side bend towards the left (fig. 2). Exhale and return. Side bend to the opposite side.

3. Repeat side bending two more times on each side. Switch the legs to the right side of the body and repeat the sequence.

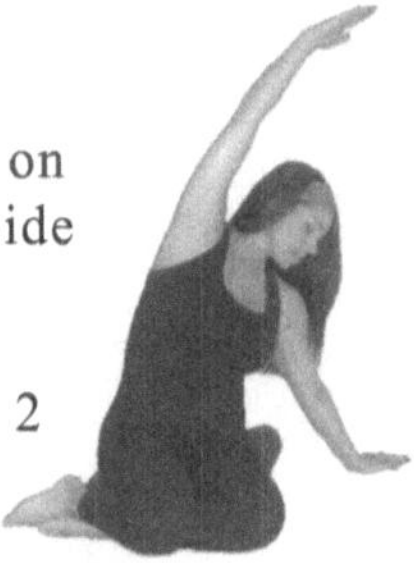

*HINT

fig. 2

Do not overstretch in this pose. Be very gentle with your body.

SEATED HALF - SPINAL TWIST

1. Begin seated onto a pillow cross-legged, or if more comfortable for you, fold your right leg underneath you and place your left leg over the right knee (fig. 1).

2. Place the left hand onto the left calf, or if sitting crossed-legged, place the left hand onto the right knee. Place the right hand behind the back. Lengthen up through the spine reaching the crown of the head toward the ceiling.

3. Inhale to prepare and as you exhale gently twist the torso towards the right as you look back behind the right shoulder. Hold for 3 breaths relaxing deeper into the posture with every exhale.

4. Cross the legs the opposite way and twist to the opposite side.

*HINT
When practicing twisting poses, twist from the shoulders and back to avoid putting any pressure on your abdomen.

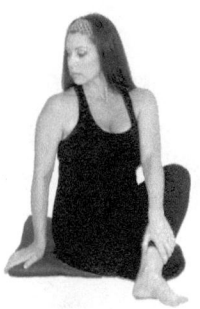

fig. 1

LYING ON THE BACK EXERCISES/POSES

SUPPORTED SHOULDER POSE

1. Lie on the back with both knees bent and the soles of the feet flat on the floor. Place a pillow beneath the buttocks. Bring the heels close into the buttocks. The feet and knees are hip width apart. Relax the hands beside the hips (fig. 1).

2. Inhale slowly and gently push the hips up into the air as far as is comfortable for you. Place the hands under the hips for support (figs. 2 & 3). Hold for a few moments. Press the feet downward into the floor and the hips upward toward the ceiling.

3. Exhale to slowly lower the body. Repeat 5 times.

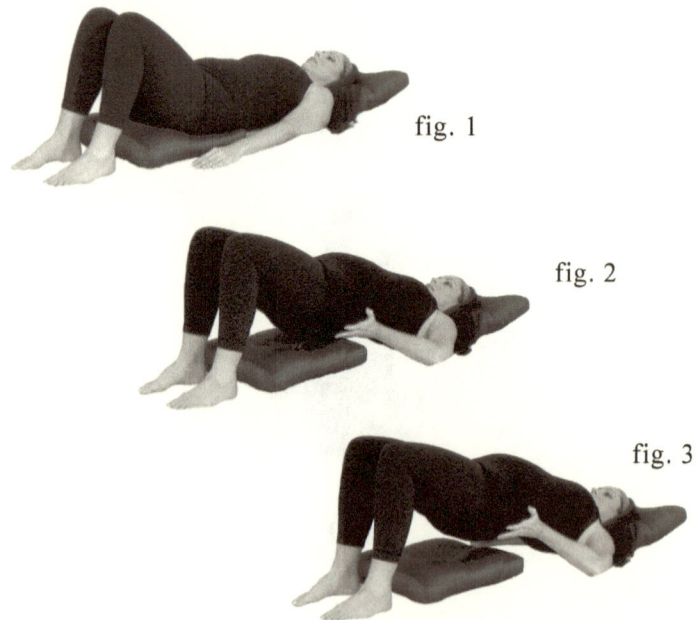

fig. 1

fig. 2

fig. 3

EASY SPINAL TWIST

1. Lie on the back with a pillow beneath the head. Bend the knees and place the feet flat onto the floor hip width apart. Reach the arms out to the sides in alignment with the shoulders. Press the palms downward into the floor.

2. Inhale to prepare and as you exhale bring both knees to the right and turn the head to the left to look over the left fingertips (fig. 1).

3. Inhale to return to the center and exhale to lower the knees to the opposite side. Turn the head to the opposite side as well. Repeat 5 times on each side. Move slowly from side to side. Press the palms into the floor for support.

fig. 1

SIDE LYING RELAXATION POSE

Lie onto the left side of the body. Place a pillow under the head. Place the left arm beneath the head and pillow. The right hand can rest onto the hip, tummy or onto the floor. Find the most comfortable position. Bend the right leg forward and rest it onto a pillow. The left leg is extended straight. Allow the eyes to close and each and every muscle in the body to rest. Focus on the breath. Take deep breaths into the nose and release any and all tension on the exhales. Exhale through the nose as well. Enjoy the peace and calm this pose brings to you and your baby. Stay in this pose as long as you'd like.

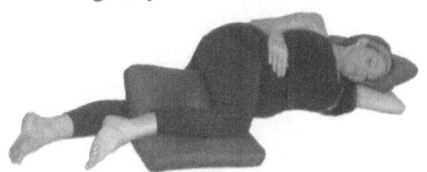

MEDITATION

WHAT IS MEDITATION?

Meditation is a mind/body medicine, and it is a means
of transforming your mind. When you are no longer
distracted by external stimuli and when your mind is
completely controlled, remaining effortlessly at one point,
that is meditation. Meditation techniques help you to
experience inner silence and peace as well as physical and
mental equilibrium. Regular practice of meditation will
induce a deep sense of rejuvenation and relaxation. By
engaging with a particular meditation practice you learn
the patterns and habits of the mind, and the practice offers
a means to cultivate new, more positive ways of being and
understanding.

WHY IS MEDITATION HELPFUL?

As far as for healing purposes, meditation can help to
resolve the deep seated fears and conflicts which can
cause stress and ill-health in the body and mind. Stress
reduction is one of the most commonly known benefits of
meditation. Meditation has been known to be a useful
technique to relieve not only stress but also pain. Meditation is helpful in dealing with anxiety, stress, depression,
and maintaining a healthy lifestyle. Meditation helps to
build self confidence, affect your moods and behavior
positively, enhances your energy levels while creating a
state of deep relaxation and general feeling of wellbeing.
Even better, the peace of mind and tranquility you'll
experience continues much further than just the time that
you actually spend meditating. Your entire day and
possibly days to follow will flow more smoothly, and
you'll be able to approach your daily routines with a sense
of ease and effortlessness.

WHY SHOULD I MEDITATE DURING PREGNANCY?

Meditation will help you to more fully "see" your inner self, and to bond and connect with your child in a way that is not possible to explain. It helps to develop an exceptional understanding of you and you alone. It allows a deep union with you and your baby. Meditation during your pregnancy can help to reduce the stress you go through as you prepare for childbirth. During pregnancy it is common to feel stressors more intensely than you normally would feel them. It is a perfect time to begin meditation because it will help you deal with the pains of labor both physically as well as mentally. The single most important thing during your labor is maintaining a sense of calm. Our bodies go through so many changes during the nine months leading up to birth that it can cause a bit of anxiety as well as many aches and pains. Meditation is a tool for you to use to combat these feelings of concern.

The more relaxed you are during actual labor you will undoubtedly experience a more comfortable childbirth because you will be flowing with your body's natural rhythms rather than fighting against them. There are many benefits to meditation and I have only touched on a few.

The most incredible benefit of meditation during your pregnancy though is the ability to deeply connect and bond with your baby and the consciousness of sensing and feeling your baby's growth and development inside your belly.

WHERE DO I MEDITATE?

Find a space in which you feel comfortable. As much as possible, this space should feel peaceful and serene to you and be free of any distractions. Be sure the temperature is just right for you. Depending on how far along you are in your pregnancy, you may find it more comfortable to begin meditating while lying down on your back or sitting up in a comfortable supported chair.

Be sure that whichever position you choose, your spine
and head are in a straight line as this will help you with
your breathing. You may also want to place a pillow
under your head or under your lower back for support if
lying on your back. If neither of these positions is comfortable, then side lying is permissible as long as you are
not so comfortable you fall to sleep.

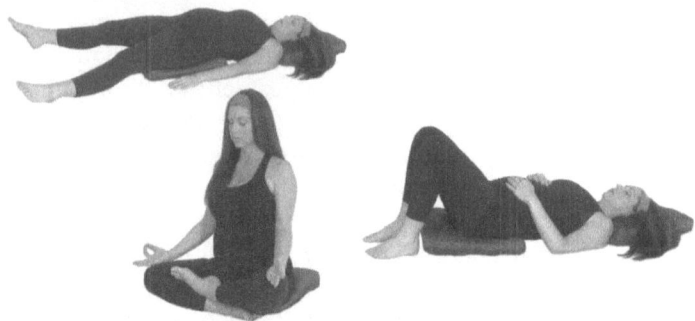

HOW TO MEDITATE

Begin by breathing deeply and slowly from your
abdomen. Inhale through your nose and exhale through
your nose. Notice and then feel your stomach rise and
fall. Then notice your rib cage expand and relax, and then
notice your chest rise and fall. Now notice all three in
unison breathing together. Take deep breaths in and
exhale for an equal amount of time. Try to consciously
relax every muscle in your body very slowly. Start first at
your toes, and then work your way up to your head as you
imagine every muscle melting until all of the tension
melts away and your body feels calm and peaceful.
Eventually you will get to place where you do not feel
your physical body at all because you will become one
with it. A peacefulness and unity overcomes you. You
may notice though that your mind wants to wander,
bouncing from thought to another. It jumps from thing
and then to the next. Try to gently bring your attention
back to a single point such as your breath until it rests
there naturally. Always come back to your breath if you

wander off. Let your attention rest on the flow of your breath. Feel the air as it comes into your nostrils and then as it leaves your nostrils. Listen to it and follow it. Beginners may find it easier to count their breaths. Try counting your breath as you inhale from 1 to 8 or 10, then exhale and count the same. Then simply start again at 1. Take your attention above all thoughts to a point you lose all attention and all thoughts. The goal is to allow the "voices" in your mind to gradually fade away and to silence your mind totally. Once you've trained your mind to focus on just one thing at a time,such as your breath, the next step is focus on nothing at all, essentially "clearing" or emptying out your mind.

What you do with a silent mind is up to you. You could then introduce an intention or a desired outcome to the subconscious mind. You could visualize a perfect birthing experience. You could meditate on a word such as peace or love. You could also just "rest" in the amazing silence and peace that your meditation brings. Experiment with a variety of ways and see what works best for you.

Try to set aside a specific time each day for meditation. Twice a day if you'd like. Start with 10 to 20 minutes and work up to longer periods of time. The more you practice, the easier it will become and your experiences will be much more profound.

CONCLUSION

I hope this book has been an inspiration to you throughout this very special time in your life. Understanding the
flow and harmony of this routine can be an amazing and
wonderful experience for you and your baby. As you
become more in tune with your body, your breath and
your movements, your quality of life will improve and
you will experience more peace. Your baby will feel the
harmony as you do. This contentment will prepare you for
the challenging new role of motherhood.

"Yoga and Pilates for your Mind, Body and Baby"
combines both yoga and pilates to give you the strength
and stamina as well as the flexibility and relaxation to
gracefully move throughout your entire pregnancy. The
more time you spend practicing these techniques the more
you will allow yourself to connect to your unborn baby.
You will learn so much about yourself the more you let
go, breathe and slow yourself down. Trust your body, feel
what you are feeling, and enjoy every moment of this
beautiful experience you are now enduring.

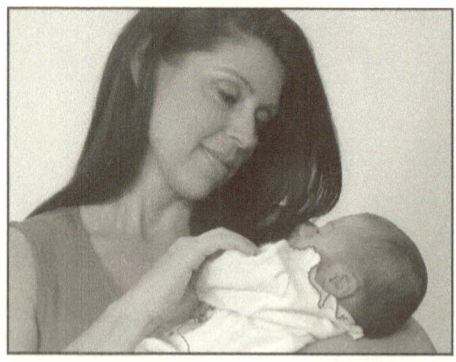

Lisa and Nina Daniel-Roth